Health Information
Management Case Studies

Second Edition

ISBN: 978-1-58426-769-0
AHIMA Product No.: AB125118

AHIMA Staff:
Jessica Block, MA, Production Development Editor
Megan Grennan, Managing Editor
James Pinnick, Senior Director of Publications
Rachel Schratz, MA, Assistant Editor

Cover image: ©shuoshu, iStock

For more information, including updates, about AHIMA Press publications, visit http://www.ahima.org/education/press.

American Health Information Management Association
233 North Michigan Avenue, 21st Floor
Chicago, Illinois 60601-5809
ahima.org

Health Information Management Case Studies

Second Edition

Dianna M. Foley, RHIA, CCS, CDIP, CHPS

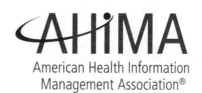

AHiMA

American Health Information
Management Association®

Brief Table of Contents

Table of Contents

Chapter 2

Chapter 3

Chapter 4

Chapter 5

Introduction

Welcome to *Health Information Management Case Studies*, Second Edition. This book supplements health information management (HIM) programs at the associate, baccalaureate, and graduate degree levels. The book can be used throughout the academic program in courses on reimbursement and coding, legal and ethics, management, privacy and security, quality and performance improvement, data management, data analysis, statistics, and more.

Every curricula competency for associate and baccalaureate programs is addressed by at least one case that meets or exceeds the Bloom's Taxonomy level required in the AHIMA 2018 Health Information Management Curricula Competencies. There are scenarios that meet the required Bloom's level for 85 percent of the curricular competencies for the graduate level.

The case studies within this book are classified by curricula competency and Bloom's level. The curricula map, found in the instructor's materials, illustrates which scenarios are applicable to each curricula competency and the Bloom's level it meets. This gives instructors the ability to choose scenarios appropriate to the program and course taught. For example, case 1.0 addresses competency I.5 and meets the Bloom's level for both associate and baccalaureate programs. For that same competency, I.5, the Bloom's level for case 1.3 also meets the graduate level, while case 1.14 is only applicable for associate-level courses.

Competency I.5:

1.0	A, B
1.3	A, B, G
1.14	A

Keep in mind, while any scenario that would meet the Bloom's level for baccalaureate or graduate programs would automatically meet (or exceed) the level for the associate degree program, it may be too advanced for beginners without appropriate preliminary work. Instructors should use their judgment when incorporating the material into coursework.

About the Author

Dianna M. Foley, RHIA, CCS, CDIP, CHPS has been an HIM professional for 20 years, holding jobs as coder, department supervisor, department director, and now as a coding consultant. She earned her bachelor's degree from the University of Cincinnati subsequently achieving her RHIA, CHPS, CCS, and CDIP certifications. Ms. Foley previously served as the program director for medical coding and HIT at Eastern Gateway Community College. She is an AHIMA-approved ICD-10-CM/PCS trainer and is the Coding Education Coordinator for OHIMA. Along with authoring this textbook, Ms. Foley co-authored *Basic ICD-10-CM and ICD-10-PCS Coding Exercises*, Sixth Edition, and was a technical editor for the 2017 edition of the *Clinical Coding Workout* book. In addition, Ms. Foley was a contributor to AHIMA's Code Update Rapid Design Project in 2016 and 2017, and as a member of AHIMA's Coding Roundtable Coordinators, she participated in updating the Coding Roundtable Coordinator's Toolkit in 2016 and 2018. Ms. Foley has also served on AHIMA's item writing, exam development, and standard setting committees. She has presented webinars for AHIMA and OHIMA on a variety of coding topics. She serves on the OHIMA board in capacities such as newsletter contributor, participant on the scholarship and awards committee, and facilitator of coding roundtables. Ms. Foley mentors new AHIMA members and provides monthly educational lectures to coders and clinical documentation specialists.

Acknowledgments

AHIMA Press would like to thank Kerry Heinecke, MS, RHIA, and Lisa Rae Roper MS, MHA, CCS-P, CPC, CPC-I, PCS, FAHIMA for their technical review of this textbook.

Dianna Foley would like to thank Robert Brzezinski, CHPS, CISA, CISM for sharing his expertise with the privacy and security case studies.

Online Resources

For Instructors

AHIMA provides supplementary materials for educators who use this book in their classes. Materials include an answer key, curriculum maps, and discussion questions. Visit **http://www .ahimapress.org/Foley7690** and click the link to download the files. If you have any questions regarding the instructor materials, contact AHIMA Customer Relations at (800) 335-5535 or submit a customer support request at https://secure.ahima.org/contact/contact.aspx.

Icon Key

The following icons appear throughout the book to indicate the academic and Bloom's Taxonomy levels of the cases and tasks within.

Associate Level
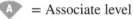

A

Baccalaureate Level
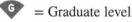

B

Graduate Level
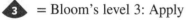

G

The tabs along the outer edge of each page are a visual aid to help locate activities by degree level. The competencies addressed are listed before each case.

A = Associate level

B = Baccalaureate level

G = Graduate level

1 = Bloom's level 1: Remember

2 = Bloom's level 2: Understand

3 = Bloom's level 3: Apply

4 = Bloom's level 4: Analyze

5 = Bloom's level 5: Evaluate

6 = Bloom's level 6: Create

One or more sets of pie piece symbols appear next to each competency. The degree level is designated by the top symbol and the Bloom's Taxonomy level is designated by the bottom symbol. The competencies listed in the book correspond to the domain of the chapter where the case is located. Additional competencies that are outside of the chapter's domain apply to some cases; these are denoted in the online instructor's key in italic font.

Chapter 1

Domain I: Data Governance, Content, and Structure

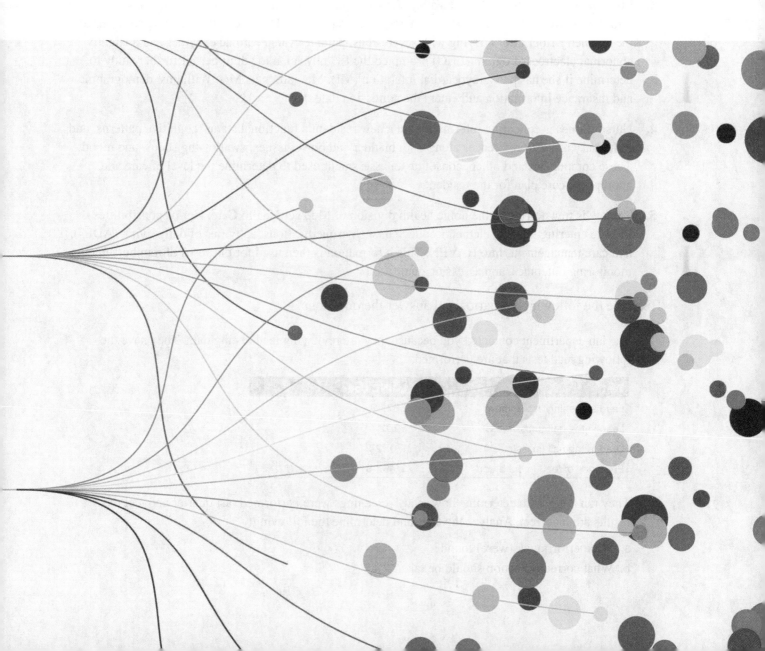

1.0   Taxonomies, nomenclatures, and terminologies

Competency I.5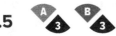

Identify the healthcare data set used in each scenario below.

1. A 42-year-old male came to the emergency department (ED) with chest pain, which has been occurring more frequently after meals in the last week. Today, the chest pressure was intense and did not ease, so the patient came to the hospital. The ED doctor ran cardiac enzymes, troponin level, and has an EKG performed, all of which return normal. The patient was diagnosed with gastroesophageal reflux disease, given a prescription for medication, and told to follow up with his family doctor in a week.

2. The human resource director of Pinewood Nursing Home is investigating a potential change to the healthcare insurance Pinewood currently provides to the staff. He is comparing several different health plans to determine their overall accreditation status and their outcomes related to asthma, diabetes, and hypertension.

3. Margaret is an admitting clerk at Valley View Hospital. She is in the process of collecting information from Mrs. Williams, an emergency department (ED) patient who is being admitted to the telemetry floor after arriving with severe chest pain. Elevated cardiac enzymes and a slightly abnormal electrocardiogram (EKG) prompted the ED physician to admit her for further study to determine if she has had a myocardial infarction (MI). Margaret gets Mrs. Williams' demographic and insurance information and enters the admission date.

4. Nurse Barnes is collecting information on a new resident's functional status, cognitive patterns, and customary routine preferences along with bladder and bowel issues, swallowing status, and mood. These components and others constitute an assessment used to determine the level of care and appropriate care plan for the resident.

5. Tammy is transferring to the home health division of Metzger Health Care. Her responsibilities include entering the data elements collected, such as medications, activities of daily living (ADLs), and care management, into HAVEN. This information is then used for purposes of reimbursement, monitoring outcomes, and assessing quality.

Examine the following scenarios and answer the questions.

1. The lab department contacted you because they are reviewing lead testing data. They have the following lead tests that are performed:

Test	LOINC Code
Lead screening assessment	5673-9
Lead in the hair (mass/mass)	8202-4
Lead in the nail (mass/mass)	17052-2
Presence of lead in the blood	39193-8

They ran a report to determine how many screenings were performed last quarter and feel the results are incorrect. Analyze the tests and determine the following:

a. What error(s) was(were) found?

b. What corrective action should be taken?

2. The classification system for cancer is based on morphology and topography.

   a. What is it called?

   b. Examine the following codes and provide the type of cancer and behavior signified.
   - M9823/3
   - M8042/3
   - M8081/2
   - M8140/0
   - M8010/6
   - M8140/1

3. The Unified Medical Language System (UMLS) is a metathesaurus. Different vocabularies are used in this resource. Consider the following types of data, and indicate the vocabulary that would be used for reporting:
   - HbA1c Laboratory Test
   - Catapres 0.1 mg tablet
   - Type II diabetes
   - Preventive Care Services, Established Office Visit, 18 and up

4. Explain why the UMLS would have been helpful during the transition from ICD-9 to ICD-10-CM.

5. Nomenclatures undergo periodic evaluation and update. Investigate how the *Diagnostic and Statistical Manual of Mental Disorders*, 5th Edition (DSM-5) impacted coding for hoarding in 2017. As part of your investigation, determine if the DSM-5 and the code set are fully aligned with this code and support your position.

6. The *Diagnostic and Statistical Manual of Mental Disorders*, 5th Edition (DSM-5) has a built-in crosswalk to what other classification system(s)?

7. Search the internet for the components of a national drug code and outline below.

8. Given the following National Drug Codes (NDC), map to the specific drug it represents and breakdown the information contained in the code for further detail.
   - 0056-0174-01
   - 0004-0186-83

9. Supply the NDC code for the following medications.
   - Xarelto 20 mg oral 90 film-coated tablets in 1 bottle Janssen Pharmaceuticals, Inc.
   - Caduet 10 mg/80 mg oral 30 film-coated tablets in 1 bottle Pfizer Laboratories

Resources

American Psychological Association (APA). 2018. https://www.psychiatry.org/psychiatrists/practice /dsm/history-of-the-dsm.

Giannangelo, K. ed. 2019. *Healthcare Code Sets, Clinical Terminologies, and Classification Systems*, 4th ed. Chicago: AHIMA.

Regenstrief Institute. 2018. LOINC Version 2.65. https://loinc.org.

World Health Organization. n.d. International Classification of Diseases for Oncology: ICD-O-3 Online. Accessed 14 June 2019. http://codes.iarc.fr.

US Food and Drug Administration (FDA). 2017. National Drug Code Directory. https://www.fda.gov /drugs/drug-approvals-and-databases/national-drug-code-directory.

US Food and Drug Administration (FDA). 2019. National Drug Code Directory. https://www.accessdata .fda.gov/scripts/cder/ndc/index.cfm.

1.1 Ambulatory surgery data collection

Competency I.2

Competency I.4

1. Northwest Ambulatory Surgery Center provides urology, endoscopy, orthopedic, otolaryngology, and ophthalmology procedures. Physicians for each service are listed here:

   Urology: Dr. Westerly, Dr. Columbia

   Endoscopy: Dr. Southcliffe, Dr. Harvard, Dr. Cornell, Dr. Penn

   Ophthalmology: Dr. Easton, Dr. Northrop

   Orthopedic: Dr. Yale, Dr. C. Princeton

   Otolaryngology: Dr. L. Princeton

In keeping with Joint Commission requirements, the center has a documentation requirement that every patient's health record must have an H&P prior to surgery. Data is being collected to verify compliance with that requirement.

   a. Determine which data elements should be included in the data collection.

   b. Create a data collection checklist to be used in the chart review.

2. In June, Northwest Ambulatory Surgery Center conducted a chart audit to determine compliance with the H&P on the chart prior to surgery requirement. The results are as follows:

   A total of 1220 surgeries were performed in May:
   640 endoscopies
   160 urological procedures
   240 ophthalmologic procedures
   120 otolaryngology procedures
   60 orthopedic procedures

100 total charts were reviewed:

Dr. Northrop	7 charts	6 with H&P	1 w/o H&P
Dr. Easton	22	22 with H&P	
Dr. Westerly	33	30 with H&P	3 w/o H&P
Dr. Southcliffe	28	20 with H&P	8 w/o H&P
Dr. Penn	10	10 with H&P	

Examine the results of the data collection and answer the following questions.

a. Upon review of the information, what can be deduced about the data collection in general?

b. Propose a more meaningful data collection.

c. What deductions can be made regarding the results of the data collection as presented above?

d. Create a graph to depict the data collection results.
e. Based only on the data collection above, create a graphic design which illustrates the missing H&Ps by service.

Resource

Shaw P. L. and D. Carter. 2019. Defining a performance improvement model. Chapter 2 in *Quality and Performance Improvement in Healthcare: A Tool for Programmed Learning*, 7th ed. Chicago: AHIMA.

1.2 International classification of diseases mapping exercise

Competency I.5

Distinguish the international classification of diseases (ICD) codes below, identifying them as ICD-9-CM, ICD-10-CM, or ICD-10-PCS. Then, map each code to its counterpart in the other classification. Provide an explanation for the mapped code assignment.

Example:	Chronic kidney disease in ICD-9 585.9 maps to N18.3 ICD-10 code—this is a one-to-one match

Example:	Closed fractured shaft of clavicle in ICD-9 810.02 maps to S42.021 (A, D, G, K, P, or S)—this is a one-to-many match

a. T38.3X6A
b. 86.4
c. E10.311
d. 91.44
e. 576.2

Resources

Centers for Disease Control and Prevention (CDC). 2019. ICD-10-CM. ftp://ftp.cdc.gov/pub /Health_Statistics/NCHS/Publications/ICD10CM/2019/.

Centers for Disease Control and Prevention (CDC). 2011. ICD-9-CM. ftp://ftp.cdc.gov/pub /Health_Statistics/NCHS/Publications/ICD9-CM/2011.

Centers for Medicare and Medicaid Services (CMS). 2019. ICD-10-CM and ICD-10 PCS and GEMs Archive. https://www.cms.gov/Medicare/Coding/ICD10/Archive-ICD-10-CM-ICD-10-PCS-GEMs. html.

1.3 Coding audit

Competency I.5

As coding supervisor, you are auditing the coding accuracy of two outpatient coders on the following orthopedic charts. You are auditing ICD-10-CM diagnoses and CPT procedures.

1. First, create an audit checklist. Decide what data elements are relevant to collect and include them in the checklist.

2. Perform the audit of the following 10 scenarios.

3. Create three different meaningful data display of the results.

4. Formulate an educational plan to address any inaccuracies found.

B

G

Op Report 1. Coder DEF   **Codes: S83.242A, 27332-LT**

Acct. # 0632175   **DOS: 2/05/16**

Pt. Name: Mr. John Jones   **Physician: Dr. M. Patrick**

PREOPERATIVE DIAGNOSIS:

Left knee medial meniscal tear

POSTOPERATIVE DIAGNOSIS:

Posterior horn tear around medial meniscus

NAME OF OPERATION:

Left knee arthroscopy with partial medial meniscectomy

ANESTHESIA: General

PROCEDURE: Patient arrived in OR and was prepped and draped in the normal method for knee surgery. Tourniquet applied and a stab incision made for the anterolateral portal. The arthroscope was then introduced via the trocar.

Examination of the suprapatellar pouch was performed first with slight chondromalacia found and debrided. I moved to the medial compartment where I found a posterior horn medial meniscus tear which I debrided back to a stable rim. Lateral compartment was examined and found to be in good shape with no abnormalities.

I removed the scope and repaired the incision sites with 4-0 nylon suture. Marcaine 0.5 percent injected into the knee for pain relief and then the patient was taken to the recovery room in stable condition.

Op report 2. Coder DEF Codes: **S38.231A, S83.271A, M22.41, 29880-RT, 29877-RT**

Acct. # 0648461 DOS: **2/15/16**

Pt. Name: Mrs. Martha Mason Physician: **Dr. J. Harris**

PREOPERATIVE DIAGNOSIS:

Meniscal tears (medial and lateral)

POSTOPERATIVE DIAGNOSIS:

Complex lateral and complex medial meniscus tears.

Patellar chondromalacia

SURGERY TO BE PERFORMED:

Lateral and medial meniscectomy.

Chondroplasty.

PROCEDURE: General anesthesia was administered once the patient was brought to the operating room. Appropriate draping of the right knee was done and then a timeout to verify the correct patient and procedure was performed.

Tourniquet was applied and an arthroscope introduced into the suprapatellar pouch where a chondroplasty of the patella for the chondromalacia that was identified was performed. I moved to the medial compartment where it was immediately evident there was a complex medial meniscus tear. I did a meniscectomy of the complex tear and then shifted focus to the lateral compartment. There another complex tear, this time of the lateral meniscus, was found. I performed a lateral meniscectomy and then withdrew the scope. Local anesthetic injection of 0.5 percent Marcaine was given to assist with pain control. Tourniquet was removed and the patient was taken to recovery in excellent condition.

Follow up in 2 weeks or earlier if any problems arise.

Op report 3. Coder DEF Codes: **S83.222A, S83.252A, M22.41, M17.12, 29870-LT, 29880-LT, 29877-LT**

Acct. # 0634899 DOS: **2/13/16**

Pt. Name: Mr. Jason Johnson Physician: **Dr. M. Patrick**

PREOP DX:

Left knee tear medial meniscus

POSTOP DX:

1. Peripheral medial meniscal tear, left
2. Bucket-handle tear lateral meniscus, left
3. Degenerative joint disease, primary, left
4. Patellar chondromalacia, left

PROCEDURE PERFORMED:

1. Diagnostic arthroscopy, left knee.
2. Medial and lateral meniscectomy, left knee.
3. Patellar chondroplasty.

ANESTHESIA:

General.

PROCEDURE: Patient brought to the OR where general anesthesia was given. After appropriate sterile prepping, portals were created medially and laterally and the arthroscope introduced into the knee for a diagnostic arthroscopy. Suprapatellar pouch investigated first where grade II chondromalacial changes were found necessitating a patellar chondroplasty. No loose bodies were found. I moved to the medial compartment and shaved the tear to achieve a smooth rim. The same technique was used on the lateral meniscus tear. The knee was then irrigated and suctioned. I injected Marcaine at 0.25 percent to help control any post-operative pain. The patient went to recovery in stable condition and will be followed in the office in three weeks.

Op report 4. Coder DEF	**Codes: S83.221A, S82.261A, 29883-RT**
Acct. # 0627765	**DOS: 2/2/16**
Pt. Name: Mr. Donald Davison	**Physician: Dr. M. Patrick**

PREOPERATIVE DIAGNOSIS:

Right knee lateral meniscus tear

POSTOPERATIVE DIAGNOSIS:

Same with medial meniscus tear (both peripheral in nature)

ANESTHESIA:

General

PROCEDURE: After arrival in the OR, general anesthesia was given to the patient. Sterile prep and drape was performed and the arthroscope was introduced into the patient's right knee. I examined the patellofemoral joint and found no evidence of disease. Moving to the medial compartment showed a peripheral tear in the medial meniscus which I repaired with two sutures. The same technique was then used on the peripheral tear of the lateral meniscus. Instrumentation was removed following irrigation and suctioning. The small portal sites were closed. Patient was then taken to post-anesthesia care unit (PACU) in good condition.

OP report 5. Coder DEF	**Codes: S83.511A, S83.281A, 29870-RT, 29888-RT, 29882-RT**
Acct. # 0646923	**DOS: 2/18/16**
Pt. Name: Miss Shirley Shields	**Physician: Dr. J. Harris**

PREOPERATIVE DIAGNOSES:

Right ACL tear

POSTOPERATIVE DIAGNOSES:

ACL tear right knee

Posterior horn lateral meniscus tear, complete, right

PROCEDURES PERFORMED:

Diagnostic arthroscopy

Right ACL reconstruction

Repair of lateral meniscus

ANESTHESIA:

General

PROCEDURE: The 28-year-old male arrived in the OR and general anesthetic was administered. His right knee was immobilized and a tourniquet applied. Appropriate sterile, prepping, and draping occurred and then the procedure was begun by harvesting the hamstring tendon. I created the portal sites and examined the knee compartments, noting no pathology in the medial compartment but a posterior horn lateral meniscus tear which I repaired with sutures.

After the knee was cleaned of loose debris, a tibial guide was used and tibial and femoral tunnels were drilled. A U-shaped guide was utilized to pull the harvested tendon up and then pinned. Cycling of the knee was then done with no impingement noted. Scope removed from the knee which was then irrigated and suctioned. The tourniquet was removed and immobilizer placed. Patient tolerated the procedure well and went to PACU in good condition. Follow-up instructions provided to spouse along with instruction to make appointment for office visit in two weeks.

Op report 6. Coder LMB	**Codes: S83.271A, S83.231A, M21.851, M32.41, 29870-RT, 29880-RT, 29879-RT, 29874-RT**
Acct. # 0631167	**DOS: 02/04/16**
Pt. Name: Mr. Carl Collins	**Physician: Dr. J. Harris**

PREOP DX:

Medial meniscus tear, right

Right osteochondral defect, distal femur

POSTOP DX:

Right medial and lateral meniscus tears complex in nature

Right osteochondral defect, distal femur

Loose bodies

OPERATIONS PERFORMED:

1. Right knee diagnostic arthroscopy, with complex medial and lateral meniscectomies.
2. Microfracture.
3. Loose body removal.
4. Extensive debridement of knee.

ANESTHESIA:

General

OPERATION: Patient arrived in OR where sterile prep and drape took place. A surgical timeout was taken prior to applying the tourniquet to the right lower extremity. The arthroscope was inserted through the portals and substantial synovitis was noted in the suprapatellar pouch which I debrided. Moving the medial compartment, loose bodies, three small ones, were identified and removed from the region. A complex tear of the medial meniscus was noted as we moved to the medial compartment. I shaved the meniscus and moved to the lateral compartment where an identical procedure was completed on the lateral meniscus. It was also evident that distal femoral area would benefit from a microfracture procedure that I performed. The knee was irrigated then and suctioned clean. Marcaine injected. The tourniquet was removed and sterile dressings applied to the knee. The patient was taken to recovery and given instructions for follow up in two weeks.

Op report 7. Coder LMB	**Codes: S83.511A, 27407-LT**
Acct. # 0631832	**DOS: 02/11/16**
Pt. Name: Mr. Kevin Kendrickson	**Physician: Dr. J. Harris**

PREOPERATIVE DIAGNOSIS:

ACL tear, left

POSTOPERATIVE DIAGNOSES:

ACL tear, left

OPERATION PERFORMED:

ACL repair with arthroscopy, left

ANESTHESIA:

General

DESCRIPTION OF OPERATION: Patient was transported to the OR. Antibiotics were given pre-operatively. A tourniquet was placed and the patient was then prepped and draped in the normal manner. I began by dissecting hamstring tendons to use in the reconstruction. Once that was accomplished, I created a port site and inserted the arthroscope performing a diagnostic arthroscopy. All three compartments were examined and no pathology found except for the ACL tear. Initially, I debrided the ACL with a shaver, and using a bur created a notchplasty. Then I used the tibial guide to make a tunnel, after which I pulled the graft back through the tunnel. I t was secured with pins and tested for impingement, none found. The graft was secured distally and then the knee was irrigated and suctioned. Post operative pain was mitigated with injection of Marcaine. Instrumentation was removed and the small incision sites were closed by suture. Dressings applied and the patient went to recovery in stable condition.

Op Report 8. Coder LMB	**Codes: S83.281A, 27403-RT**
Acct. # 0641919	**DOS: 02/16/16**
Pt. Name: Miss Rita Reynolds	**Physician: Dr. M. Patrick**

PREOP DX:

Lateral meniscus tear, right

POSTOP DX:

Lateral meniscus tear, right

OPERATION:

Arthroscopy right knee, lateral repair

ANESTHESIA:

General

DESCRIPTION OF OPERATION: Patient arrived in the OR, and was then prepped and draped in sterile manner. Preoperative IV antibiotics were administered and general anesthesia given. Surgical timeout taken. Portal established and suprapatellar pouch examined and found to be clean. Medial compartment was examined next with no disease found. The lateral compartment was found to contain a tear which was suture-repaired. Instrumentation was removed; knee irrigated and suctioned. Marcaine injected for postoperative pain management. Portal sites closed and tourniquet removed. Patient taken to PACU in good condition.

OP Report 9. Coder LMB   **Codes: S83.511A, S83.212A, 29870-LT, 29888-LT, 29881-LT**

Acct. # 0627345   **DOS: 02/01/16**

Pt. Name: Mr. Mark Monroe   **Physician: Dr. J. Harris**

PREOPERATIVE DIAGNOSIS:

Left ACL tear

POSTOPERATIVE DIAGNOSES:

Left ACL tear

Left, medial meniscus tear, bucket-handle variety

OPERATIONS:

Left, diagnostic arthroscopy

Left, ACL repair

Left, medial meniscus repair

DESCRIPTION OF OPERATION: After the patient's arrival in the OR, a surgical timeout was taken, followed by prep and drape of knee, and administration of general anesthesia. Hamstring tendons were harvested, port sites opened, and then scope inserted. The suprapatellar pouch had no pathology on examination. Medial compartment had a bucket-handle tear which was repairable with sutures. The lateral compartment exhibited no disease processes, so I began the ACL repair performing a notchplasty. A guide was used and followed by tibial tunnel reaming. Guidewire affixed to the graft and pulled back through the tunnel, pinning it in place. I pinned the graft distally after no impingement was found through cycling. The procedure was terminated. Instruments were removed, and irrigation and suctioning done. Postoperative pain was mitigated with Marcaine injection. Sterile dressings were wrapped around the knee and then we released the tourniquet. I sent the patient to the recovery room in excellent condition.

OP Report 10. Coder LMB   **Codes: S83.231A, S83.281A, 27333-RT**

Acct. # 0631864   **DOS: 02/11/16**

Pt. Name: Mrs. Leona Leonard   **Physician: Dr. J. Harris**

PREOP DX:

Right knee pain.

POSTOP DX:

Tears medial and lateral meniscus

OPERATIONS PERFORMED:

Meniscectomy, medial and lateral

ANESTHESIA: General.

DESCRIPTION OF OPERATION: Patient arrived in OR and given IV antibiotics pre-operatively. Sterile prepping and draping was done. A tourniquet was applied to the patient's leg and the procedure was begun. Portal sites were created and the scope inserted. The suprapatellar pouch showed no evidence of pathology. The medial compartment exhibited a complex tear of the meniscus which had to be shaved. I discovered a lateral meniscus tear upon moving to examination of that compartment. Again, I shaved the meniscus. With no other pathology found, I irrigated and suctioned the knee, and then removed the instruments. The small portal sites were closed with sutures and Marcaine injected for pain relief. The patient went to recovery in good condition.

Resources

American Medical Association (AMA). 2019. *CPT Professional Edition*. Chicago: AMA.

Edgerton, C. 2020. Healthcare Statistics. Chapter 15 in *Health Information Management: Concepts, Principles, and Practice*, 6th ed. P. Oachs and A. Watters, eds. Chicago: AHIMA.

Handlon, L. 2020. Reimbursement Methodologies. Chapter 8 in *Health Information Management: Concepts, Principles, and Practice*, 6th ed. P. Oachs and A. Watters, eds. Chicago: AHIMA.

1.4 Trauma registry audit

Competency I.3

Competency I.6

As HIM supervisor at Valley View Hospital, you are conducting a trauma registry audit. You are auditing only the following data elements:

- Transport mode for arrival
- Sex
- Work related

- Emergency department discharge disposition
- Airbag deployment

- Alcohol screen

1. One of the records you have chosen to audit is listed below. Use this ED report and the Ohio Trauma Registry data dictionary to compare the results and determine accuracy of the data reported.

CC: Closed head injury

HPI: A 34-year-old female was delivering the mail when she lost control of her car on ice and hit a tree. The woman said that she was fully conscious throughout the event; however, the ambulance EMTs tell a different story. They indicate that she was unconscious for at least two minutes after their arrival on the scene as they worked to remove her from the three-point restraints. The airbag did not deploy despite the cracked windshield. The young woman remained stable during transport, although she complained of a severe right-sided temporal headache accompanied by some blurred vision.

PMH: Hypertension.

ROS: All systems reviewed and negative unless otherwise noted in the physical exam. Patient has no known allergies.

MEDICATIONS: Lisinopril.

PHYSICAL EXAMINATION:

VITALS: Blood pressure 142/88, pulse 95, respirations 22, temperature 97.9°.

HEENT: Contusion over right temporal area.

NECK: Tender on the right side.

CHEST: Tender on the right.

LUNGS: Clear.

ABDOMEN: Flat, nontender.

BACK: Tender in the c-spine area.

PELVIS: Normal.

EXTREMITIES: Contusion right thigh.

RECTAL: Not performed.

NEUROLOGIC: Patient intact.

LABORATORY DATA: Hematocrits 42.9, and 41.7. WBC 8.5. Blood alcohol level: 0.00. Urinalysis: normal. PT 13.0, PTT 31. Chemistry normal.

X-rays: C-spine, LS- spine, and pelvis x-rays completed and all returned as normal. X-ray of chest shows 1 broken rib on the right. Right distal clavicle fracture noted.

ASSESSMENT:

1. Concussion.

2. Rib fracture

3. Fracture right clavicle.

PLAN: Admit the patient to the ortho service for treatment of fractures and have trauma follow for the concussion.

Data Element	Reported Value	Audit finding
Transport Mode for Arrival	4	
Sex	1	
Work related	2	
ED discharge disposition	1	
Airbag deployment	1	
Alcohol screen	1	

Resources

Brinda, D. 2020. Data Management. Chapter 6 in *Health Information Technology: An Applied Approach,* 6th ed. N. B. Sayles and L. Gordon, eds. Chicago: AHIMA.

Ohio Trauma Registry. 2018. Trauma Acute Care Registry Data Dictionary. https://www.ems.ohio.gov/links/ems_OTR-TACR-Data-Dictionary-2019.pdf.

Sharp, M. and C. Madlock-Brown. 2020. Data Management. Chapter 6 in *Health Information Management: Concepts, Principles, and Practice*, 6th ed. P. Oachs and A. Watters, eds. Chicago: AHIMA.

1.5 Secondary data

Competency I.3

1. Specialized data collection systems, like those for cancer or trauma registries, may utilize edits to ensure data validity. Consider that you are training to become a trauma registrar in Mayfield, Ohio.
   a. Determine what validation checks will be available to you as you complete your data collection entries for the mandatory state trauma reporting on-line.
   b. Identify the source document for your responses.

Resources

Ohio Trauma Registry. 2014. Web Entry Training Manual. http://www.ems.ohio.gov/links/EMS-Acute-Care-Training-Manual.pdf.

Sharp, M. and C. Madlock-Brown. 2020. Data Management. Chapter 6 in *Health Information Management: Concepts, Principles, and Practice*, 6th ed. P. Oachs and A. Watters, eds. Chicago: AHIMA.

Sharp, M. 2020. Secondary Data Sources. Chapter 7 in *Health Information Technology: An Applied Approach,* 6th ed. N. B. Sayles and L. Gordon, eds. Chicago: AHIMA.

1.6 Emergency department documentation

Competency I.2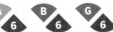

Competency I.4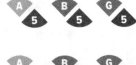

1. The emergency department (ED) chair has asked for a documentation audit of ED records. Your staff conducted the audit, the results of which were very poor. There was no consistency in the ED record documentation. You check the medical staff by-laws and realize that there are no specific guidelines related to ED documentation.

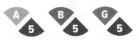

   a. Determine documentation requirements for ED reports. List them here.

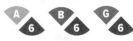

   b. Audit the five representative ED cases below to determine the major areas in need of documentation improvement. As HIM director, present your results in a short memo to the ED department chair, Dr. Wilkerson.

   c. Create a new section for the medical staff by-laws that incorporates ED documentation requirements. Include this in the memo to the chief of the ED for his approval before it continues through the formal process for inclusion into the by-laws.

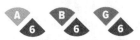

   d. The timing for this coincides with the transition of ED documentation into an electronic format. You propose to utilize the electronic record to facilitate the appropriate data collection. Create a screen design that encompasses the required ED documentation data elements.

ED Report 1:

HPI: Four-year-old female arrived after fall on trampoline. Patient fell and landed on her right elbow. Complaining of pain. Tearful.

PMH: Child currently on antibiotics for an acute otitis media infection of her left ear. Tympanum still inflamed.

IMMUNIZATIONS: Up-to-date.

ALLERGIES: None known.

PHYSICAL EXAMINATION:

VITAL SIGNS: Temperature 36.8 Celsius, pulse 95, respirations 22, blood pressure 114/77, weight 18 kilograms.

GENERAL: Alert, minimal distress upon palpation of elbow.

SKIN: Negative

HEENT: Head: Normal. Eyes: PERRL. Nose and throat normal. Ears: Left tympanum inflamed.

NECK: Supple, no lymphadenopathy, no masses.

LUNGS: Clear bilaterally.

HEART: Normal S1, S2. Regular rate.

ABDOMEN: Soft, non-tender. Bowel sounds are present.

EXTREMITIES: Warm. Right elbow tender to palpation.

NEUROLOGICAL: Alert.

X-RAY: Right elbow shows supracondylar fracture.

EMERGENCY DEPARTMENT COURSE: Patient had an x-ray of the right upper extremity which showed a displaced supracondylar fracture. A long arm splint was applied. No lab work was done.

DX: Displaced, right supracondylar fracture.

DISPOSITION: Home with parents.

ED Report 2:

CHIEF COMPLAINT: Ankle pain.

HISTORY OF PRESENT ILLNESS: A 67-year-old female fell off a curb while crossing the street. Complains of pain in left ankle and right wrist, as she landed on the wrist when she fell. No other injuries are apparent.

PMH: COPD. Hypertension. Diabetes. Smoker.

PAST SURGICAL HISTORY: Appendectomy 10 years ago.

SOCIAL HISTORY: Denies alcohol.

ALLERGIES: No known allergies.

MEDICATIONS: Spiriva. Lisinopril. Humulin.

ROS: Ten systems reviewed and negative unless noted above.

PHYSICAL EXAMINATION:

VITAL SIGNS: Temperature 98.7, pulse 81, respirations 19, blood pressure 130/83, and pulse oximetry 93 percent on room air.

GENERAL: No acute distress.

EXTREMITIES: Full range of motion in his right knee. Palpation of the ankle and Achilles tendon elicit no pain. Pulses are intact, with strong capillary refill. Normal sensation. There is pain on the lateral aspect of the right foot. Contusion and swelling noted as well. Dorsal foot pain present too.

X-RAY: Left ankle shows lateral malleolus fracture. Right wrist film shows an intraarticular distal radius fracture.

DX: Fractures of left ankle and right wrist as evidenced on x-rays. Contusion of lower left leg.

DISPOSITION: Splints applied on both extremities (arm and leg) and prescription given for Motrin 800mg. to be taken four times a day. Home to follow with ortho tomorrow.

ED Report 3:

CHIEF COMPLAINT: Shortness of breath brings this 72-year-old Caucasian female to the ED transported by her husband.

HPI: Patient is in ED often due to her COPD exacerbations. Today the patient experienced severe respiratory distress. Her husband states the patient was admitted two weeks ago with bronchial pneumonia and discharged last week. Patient continued to have a chronic cough after discharge and today all her symptoms worsened.

PMH: Hypertension, emphysema, and lupus.

MEDICATIONS: Dyazide, and Atrovent inhaler.

ALLERGIES: No known allergies.

SOCIAL HISTORY: The patient is florist, married, with 2 children.

REVIEW OF SYSTEMS: Ten system review normal except as noted above.

PHYSICAL EXAMINATION:

VITAL SIGNS: Temperature 101.3. Pulse 91. Respirations 22. Blood pressure 136/88. Initial oxygen saturations on room air are 84.

LUNGS: Auscultation of the chest reveals faint breath sounds, on the right, no obvious rales.

GENERAL: Breathing is labored.

HEART: Sinus tachycardia.

HEENT: Head is normal.

ABDOMEN: Nontender.

NECK: The neck is supple.

EXTREMITIES: Slight pedal edema.

DIAGNOSTIC DATA: White blood count 16.5, hemoglobin 15, hematocrit 41.3, Sodium of 137, chloride 80, CO2 45, BUN 7, creatinine 0.8, glucose 192, albumin 3.4 and globulin 4.0. Urinalysis normal.

X-RAY: Early infiltrates noted on chest x-ray.

EMERGENCY DEPARTMENT COURSE: One gram of Rocephin was administered intravenously as there is evidence that pneumonia is persisting. Further medication orders included Atrovent q. 2h. and Levaquin 500 mg IV. Patient appears to have a degree of respiratory failure and possible sepsis.

FINAL DIAGNOSIS: Pneumonia.

DISCHARGE INSTRUCTIONS: Patient admitted to medical floor. Will require close observation and care.

ED Report 4:

CHIEF COMPLAINT: Abdominal pain.

HPI: This 58-year-old Caucasian complains of unrelenting right lower quadrant abdominal pain. Began in the early hours of the morning, actually awakening the patient from his sleep. Has not abated and patient decided to come to ED for evaluation.

PMH: Healthy.

REVIEW OF SYSTEMS: Nausea with one episode of emesis after arrival in ED.

SOCIAL HISTORY: Married, no children.

FAMILY HISTORY: Negative.

MEDICATIONS: None.

ALLERGIES: No known allergies.

PHYSICAL EXAMINATION: VITAL SIGNS: Temperature 100.5, heart rate 95, blood pressure 125/76, respiratory rate 21. GENERAL: Patient in acute abdominal distress. HEENT: Unremarkable. NECK: Supple. LUNGS: Clear. CARDIAC: Slight tachycardia. ABDOMEN: Soft, tender at McBurney's point.

ED COURSE: Lab work done which resulted in elevated white count. Abdominal CT scan done which supported diagnosis of appendicitis.

IMPRESSION: Acute appendicitis.

ASSESSMENT AND PLAN: Admit patient and take to surgery for appendectomy. Surgeon on call notified of admission.

ED Report 5:

HPI: A 32-year-old black male arrived in the ED. He was incoherent and barely able to stand. Companion states he may have "gotten some bad drugs." Companion indicates patient did heroin 45 minutes ago and had a bad reaction, so he brought him here.

ALLERGIES: No known allergies.

MEDICATIONS: Unknown.

PAST SURGICAL HISTORY: Unknown.

FAMILY HISTORY: Unknown.

SOCIAL HISTORY: Smokes, consumes 6 beers a day, uses street drugs.

PHYSICAL EXAMINATION:

VITAL SIGNS: temperature of 99.2 degrees, pulse 66, respiratory rate is 14, and blood pressure is 90/51, recheck blood pressure was 90/50.

GENERAL: Disoriented.

HEENT: Pupils dilated.

NECK: Supple.

CHEST: Clear.

HEART: Regular.

ABDOMEN: Soft.

SKIN: Color is normal.

EXTREMITIES: Laxity in all extremities.

NEUROLOGIC: Decreased reflex responses.

ED COURSE: Labs were drawn and IV fluids started. Narcan was administered and patient had good response. Patient admitted to ICU in critical condition.

IMPRESSION: Heroin overdose.

Resources

Brickner, M. 2020. Health Record Content and Documentation. Chapter 4 in *Health Information Technology: An Applied Approach,* 6th ed. N. B. Sayles and L. Gordon, eds. Chicago: AHIMA.

Reynolds, R. B. and A. Morey. 2020. Health Record Content and Documentation. Chapter 4 in *Health Information Management: Concepts, Principles, and Practice*, 6th ed. P. Oachs and A. Watters, eds. Chicago: AHIMA.

1.7 Health information exchange data stewardship and integrity

Competency I.3

Competency I.6

1. You have just been hired as the HIM director at a 465-bed hospital. In preparation for participation in a regional health information exchange (HIE), your predecessor had just completed data collection on duplicate entries in the MPI. She found a one percent duplication rate on 21,000 registrations last month. She found that rate acceptable. You interpret the findings differently. Explain your interpretation, and assess what the next steps should be.

2. The hospital mentioned in the previous scenario serves a large population of immigrants. You discover that, as a result of a language barrier, the registration staff often searches for patients in the ADT system by date of birth rather than name. You observed this process and realized that most of the duplicates are arising from this process, as the dates of birth are not always entered correctly. Decide what other criteria the staff should search by if they do not search by date of birth only. Create a priority list of the criteria.

References

Reynolds, R. B. and A. Morey. 2020. Health Record Content and Documentation. Chapter 4 in *Health Information Management: Concepts, Principles, and Practice*, 6th ed. P. Oachs and A. Watters, eds. Chicago: AHIMA.

Sayles, N. B. 2020. Health Information Functions, Purpose, and Users. Chapter 3 in *Health Information Technology: An Applied Approach*, 6th ed. N. B. Sayles. and L. Gordon, eds. Chicago: AHIMA.

1.8 Master patient index data analysis

Competency I.3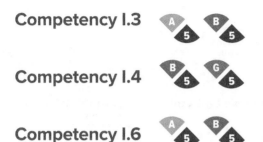

Competency I.4

Competency I.6

A

B

G

1. Study the master patient index (MPI) screen design that follows. All of the entries are for the same person. Deduce from the screen how the patient could have ended up with multiple MPI entries. Then explain the type of MPI error that has occurred and the importance of correcting these errors.

Search   ○ All Patients ○ Current Patients ○ My Patients ● MPI

Search by | Patient Name   ⬇

Birth date
Social Security Number
Medical Record Number
Admit date

Pt. Name	MR Number	Date of Birth	Social Security Number	Admit Date
Gray, Kate Ann	073251	10/12/1968	123–45–5533	07/09/2015
Gray, Karthryn Ann	021485	10/12/1968	123–45–5533	02/07/2015
Black, Kathryn Ann	154360	10/12/1968	123–45–5533	10/15/2015
Black, Kathryn Ann	159667	10/21/1968	123–45–5533	11/16/2015

2. Assume that the registration staff enters a patient by the name of Ann K. Black and mistakenly assigns her the same medical record number (154360) as Kathryn Ann Black. Which type of MPI error is this, and what issues may result from this type of error?

Resources

Reynolds, R. B. and A. Morey. 2020. Health Record Content and Documentation. Chapter 4 in *Health Information Management: Concepts, Principles, and Practice*, 6th ed. P. Oachs and A. Watters, eds. Chicago: AHIMA.

Sayles, N. B. 2020. Health Information Functions, Purpose, and Users. Chapter 3 in *Health Information Technology: An Applied Approach,* 6th ed. N. B. Sayles and L. Gordon, eds. Chicago: AHIMA.

1.9 Screen design evaluation

Competency I.3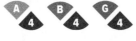

Competency I.6

Study the screen design that follows. This design was to facilitate data collection for immunizations.

Immunization Record

Patient Name	Date Vaccine given
Gender	Address
Vaccine given	Date of Birth
Lot Number	Phone number
Age	Height
Weight	Hair color
Eye color	

Additional consideration
High risk
First responder
Pregnant
Chronic medical condition
Health care worker

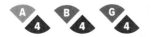

1. Identify the design flaws.

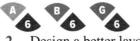

2. Design a better layout.

Resources

Amatayakul, M. 2017. Information Technology. Chapter 7 in *Health IT and EHRs Principles and Practice*, 6th ed. Chicago: AHIMA.

Brickner, M. 2020. Health Record Content and Documentation. Chapter 4 in *Health Information Management Technology: An Applied Approach*, 6th ed. N. B. Sayles and L. Gordon, eds. Chicago: AHIMA.

Sayles, N. B. 2020. Health Information Functions, Purpose, and Users. Chapter 3 in *Health Information Technology: An Applied Approach,* 6th ed. N. B. Sayles and L. Gordon, eds. Chicago: AHIMA.

1.10 Providers, roles, and documentation

Competency I.1

Competency I.2

1. A 50-year-old woman has been experiencing a chronic cough for the past two months. She is a two pack a day smoker and has been for the past 30 years. She sees her PCP for the cough and is given an order for a chest x-ray at the local hospital. The x-ray report states "nodule in lower lobe of right lung, worrisome for malignancy." The PCP refers her for a biopsy of the nodule at the ambulatory surgery clinic, which substantiates the diagnosis of cancer in the pathology report. Two weeks later, the same physician who did the biopsy performs a right lower lobectomy. Prior to discharge after surgery, the patient develops an infection, and the infectious disease specialist is asked to evaluate her and recommend the appropriate treatment course. Upon discharge, she receives care in her home for the next two weeks. Four weeks after surgery, radiation therapy is initiated, but her condition continues to deteriorate over the next few months with metastasis to the brain noted, at which point she decides to receive only palliative care.
   a. Classify the providers for each stage of the patient's care noted above and outline their responsibilities.
   b. Explain the documentation that each provider will be creating as part of the patient's record.

Resources

Fuller, S. 2020. The US Healthcare Delivery System. Chapter 1 in *Health Information Management: Concepts, Principles, and Practice,* 6th ed. P. Oachs and A. Watters, eds. Chicago: AHIMA.

Kellogg, D. 2020. Healthcare Delivery Systems. Chapter 2 in *Health Information Technology: An Applied Approach,* 6th ed. N. B. Sayles and L. Gordon, eds. Chicago: AHIMA.

A

B

1.11 Health record completion

Competency I.2

Competency I.4

1. As an HIM chart analyst, you are reviewing the chart of a patient who was admitted on 2/17 with gallstone pancreatitis. She arrived through the emergency department on Wednesday afternoon in severe abdominal pain. After lab work was performed showing an increased lipase level, she was admitted. Her family physician evaluated her the next morning and ordered an ultrasound and repeat lab work. The ultrasound showed gallstones, and the lab work indicated the lipase was coming down. He consulted a general surgeon, who evaluated the patient and agreed to perform a cholecystectomy on Friday if the lipase level returned to near normal levels. Surgery was then performed on Friday morning, and after an uneventful night, the patient was discharged home on Saturday morning. On 2/25, you have the following documentation available in the EHR:

H&P	dictated 2/18	authenticated 2/18
Consultation report	dictated 2/18	authenticated 2/23
Immediate post-op note	written 2/19	authenticated 2/19
Operative report	dictated 2/20	authenticated 2/21
Discharge summary	dictated 2/22	authenticated
Lab work from all dates of stay		
Nursing notes from all dates of stay		
Anesthesia documentation from surgery		
Physician orders from all dates of stay all signed		
Progress notes—all signed		
Medication list—signed		

At your facility, the guidelines for record completion are as follows:
- ED reports within 24 hours
- H&Ps within 24 hours of admission
- Operative reports within 24 hours of the procedure with a post-op note present immediately after the procedure
- Consultation reports within 48 hours
- Discharge summary within 14 days

1. Determine whether the record is complete or not and provide support for your answer.

2. When a record is deemed incomplete, what steps must be taken to get the record completed?

Resource

Sayles, N. B. 2020. Health Information Functions, Purpose, and Users. Chapter 3 in *Health Information Management Technology: An Applied Approach*, 6th ed. N. B. Sayles and L. Gordon, eds. Chicago: AHIMA.

1.12 Master patient index integrity

Competency I.2

Competency I.2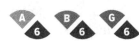

Analyze the master patient index report that follows.

a. What is the main observation from your analysis?

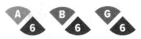

b. Create a policy that can address the issue you discovered.

MRN	SSN	Last Name	First Name	Middle	DOB	Payment
47233	546-23-XXXX	Baker Sr.	Louis	Howard	5/18/1954	Medicaid
158237	315-24-XXXX	Watson	Michelle	Lee	7/22/1942	Medicare
520613	588-32-XXXX	Jones	Lynn	Tara	10/12/1963	Commercial
723341	213-22-XXXX	Harris	Ann	Marie	9/10/1952	Self
894231	588-32-XXXX	Jones	Tara	Lynn	10/21/1963	Commercial
189011	533-44-XXXX	Marshall	Tucker	B.	11/4/1961	Commercial
218220	151-24-XXXX	Leonard	Timothy	Allen	6/17/1943	Medicare
797536	213-22-XXXX	Harris-Smythe	Ann	Marie	9/10/1952	Commercial
36524	315-24-XXXX	Watson	Michelle	Lee	7/22/1924	Medicare
466100	546-23-XXXX	Baker	Louis	Howard	5/18/1945	Medicare
744183	626-26-XXXX	Baker	Louis	Howard	4/18/1965	Commercial
118231	641-58-XXXX	Thomas	Paul	Carlson	1/16/1971	Self
237352	641-58-XXXX	Carlson	Thomas	Paul	1/16/1971	Self
898233	213-22-XXXX	HarrisSmythe	Ann	Marie	9/1/1952	Commercial
789321	151-24-XXXX	Allen	Timothy	Leonard	6/17/1934	Medicare
664455	213-22-XXXX	SmytheHarris	Ann	Marie	9/1/1925	Commercial
98723	315-42-XXXX	Watson	Michelle	Lee	7/22/1924	Medicare
587532	546-23-XXXX	Baker	Howard	Louis	5/18/1954	Medicaid

Resources

Reynolds, R. B. and A. Morey. 2020. Health Record Content and Documentation. Chapter 4 in *Health Information Management*: Concepts, Principles, and Practice, 6th ed. P. Oachs and A. Watters, eds. Chicago: AHIMA.

Sayles, N. B. 2020. Health Information Functions, Purpose, and Users. Chapter 3 in Health Information Management Technology: *An Applied Approach*, 6th ed. N. B. Sayles and L. Gordon, eds. Chicago: AHIMA.

1.13 Patient-generated health data

Competency I.6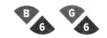

The physician you work for is concerned about incorporating patient generated health data (PGHD) into his electronic health record (EHR). Help him design a policy that not only addresses his concerns but also employs sound data stewardship principles.

a. For the purpose of this exercise, formulate a list of the topics that should be covered.

b. Create a policy.

Resources

AHIMA. 2015. Including patient-generated health data in electronic health records. *Journal of AHIMA* 86(2): 54–57.

Fountain, V. 2014. Using data provenance to manage patient-generated health data. *Journal of AHIMA* 85(11): 28–30.

LeBlanc, M. M. 2020. Human Resources Management. Chapter 22 in *Health Information Management: Concepts, Principles, and Practice*, 6th ed. P. Oachs and A. Watters, eds. Chicago: AHIMA.

1.14 Assign MS-DRG and APC groupings

Competency I.5

Kim is an HIM instructor at a local community college where she teaches courses related to coding and reimbursement. Last semester, students had trouble with the concept of how coding impacts MS-DRG assignment, so she had created the following examples to illustrate the concept. This semester, the issue is how and when it is appropriate to bypass an edit related to CPT coding and APCs. Follow the instructions given to gain a deeper understanding of these coding and reimbursement concepts.

1. Identify the MS-DRG for the following scenario:

    A 78-year-old female is discharged home with the following diagnoses:

    > Principal Dx—acute systolic, CHF

    > Additional Dx—Lupus (SLE), Insulin-dependent type 1 diabetes—uncontrolled

    MS-DRG_____

2. If the same patient also had a diagnosis of an acute exacerbation of COPD, what is the MS-DRG?

    MS-DRG_____

3. If the patient in the first example also had a diagnosis of gram negative pneumonia, what is the MS-DRG?

    MS-DRG_____

4. Now, consider that the same patient in the first scenario had to have a total system, open biventricular pacemaker inserted in the chest while admitted, with leads into the right atrium and ventricle inserted percutaneously. What MS-DRG do you get now?

    MS-DRG_____

5. A 72-year-old male has an ESWL performed for a right renal calculus. At the same operative session, the same physician removes a malignant lesion from his back resulting in a 3 cm. defect and performs an intermediate repair.
    a. Provide the CPT codes that should be assigned for this case along with their corresponding APC.
    b. When this case is coded using the encoder, an edit is given. Explain the edit.
    c. Identify if you should bypass the edit and, if so, the step(s) that would be required.

Resources

American Medical Association. 2019. *CPT Professional Edition*. Chicago: AMA.

Centers for Disease Control and Prevention (CDC). 2019. ICD-10-CM. https://www.cdc.gov/nchs/icd/icd10cm.htm.

Centers for Medicare and Medicaid Services (CMS). 2019a. ICD-10-PCS. https://www.cms.gov/Medicare/Coding/ICD10/2019-ICD-10-PCS.html.

Centers for Medicare and Medicaid Services (CMS). 2019b. Hospital Outpatient Addendum B. https://www.cms.gov/Medicare/Medicare-Fee-for-Service-Payment/HospitalOutpatientPPS/Addendum-A-and-Addendum-B-Updates-Items/2019-January-Addendum-B.html?DLPage=1&DLEntries=10&DLSort=2&DLSortDir=descending.

1.15 Special health record documentation requirements

Competency I.4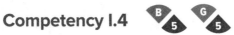

1. You have been asked to audit a pediatric group's medical records. In addition to verifying the appropriate E&M code assigned, you are tasked with ensuring that all relevant documentation is present in the record.
   a. Use the scenario and checklist that follow to determine if all relevant documentation is present in the record including discharge status.
   b. Verify the E&M code assigned. If the code is incorrect, select the appropriate code. Defend your selection whether you determine it is correct or incorrect.

OFFICE NOTE: 7/15/19

Timothy is a nine-month-old male who presents today with bilateral earaches. Timothy's mother states that the child has been crying and pulling at his ears for the last two days. She has also noticed a mild fever. Otoscopic examination revealed bulging tympanic membranes indicative of fluid buildup. Amoxicillin prescribed for ear infection. Script e-faxed to pharmacy.

CPT code assignment for visit: 99202

BIRTH HISTORY

10/09/18 Timothy had an uneventful, full-term, vaginal birth. Uncomplicated pregnancy, natural childbirth. No forceps used in delivery. APGAR score at birth 8, repeat APGAR 10.

PERSONAL, SOCIAL, AND FAMILY HISTORY

11/10/18 Second child, one older sister who is four years old. Parents are married. Non-smoking environment. No pets in the home. Will attend daycare after mother's maternity leave ends in three months. Circumsized prior to discharge at birth.

NUTRITIONAL HISTORY

11/10/18 Timothy is breastfed initially.

12/13/18 Breastfeeding continues.

2/16/19 Breastfeeding continues.

4/18/19 Cereal has been introduced into diet, rice.

7/15/19 Infant eats rice and oatmeal cereal, variety of fruits. No reactions noted to new foods.

OFFICE NOTE: 11/10/18

Well-child visit. No problems. Child thriving. Growth appropriate.

OFFICE NOTE: 12/13/18

Well-child visit. No problems. Growth appropriate. First set of vaccines administered.

OFFICE NOTE: 2/16/19

Well-child visit. No problems. Growth appropriate. Developmental milestones met. Second set of vaccines administered.

OFFICE NOTE: 4/18/19

Well-child visit. No problems. Growth appropriate. Developmental milestones met. Third set of vaccines administered.

MEDICATIONS

   7/15/19 Amoxicillin BID for 10 days.

CHECKLIST

   ☐ Office note—well-child or medical issue

   ☐ Birth history

   ☐ Nutritional history

   ☐ Personal, social, and family history

   ☐ Growth and development record

   ☐ Immunizations

   ☐ Medications

   ☐ Discharge status

Resources

American Medical Association. 2019. *CPT Professional Edition*. Chicago: AMA.

Brickner, M. R. 2020. Health Record Content and Documentation. Chapter 4 in *Health Information Management Technology: An Applied Approach*, 6th ed. N. B. Sayles and L. Gordon, eds. Chicago: AHIMA.

1.16 Physician assistant documentation practices

Competency I.1

Rockville Family Practice in Florida is considering hiring physician assistants (PA). The physicians need some clarification on the scope of work permitted by law and want you, their HIM manager, to find the answers to several questions. You identify the following website as a resource to find the answers: http://www.bartonassociates.com/nurse-practitioners/physician-assistant-scope-of-practice-laws/.

1. Research the questions and provide your conclusions to the physicians in a memo.
   a. Is there a limit to the number of PAs that can be supervised by a physician?

   b. Can a PA write prescriptions?

   c. Are the physicians required to co-sign PA documentation?

2. Do some further research and answer the following questions.
   a. Compare the results for the same questions for Florida with those from Texas, Arkansas, and West Virginia. Outline the differences in a table.

   b. Offer an opinion for why some states limit the number of PAs physicians can supervise.

   c. As an HIM manager, critique the following co-signature requirement: Records will be co-signed in a timely manner.

Resource

Barton Associates. 2019. Physician Assistant Scope of Practice Laws. http://www.bartonassociates.com/nurse-practitioners/physician-assistant-scope-of-practice-laws/.

1.17 Interoperability and SNOMED CT

Competency I.5

As an HIM professional who was just hired by a health information exchange (HIE), you have realized that although you are very familiar working with classification systems like ICD-10, you have little knowledge about the SNOMED-CT terminology and the role it plays for HIEs. Explain the reasons behind the usage of SNOMED-CT for interoperability; then, identify at least four ways that SNOMED-CT facilitates patient care.

Resources

Giannangelo, K. 2020. Clinical Terminologies, Classifications, and Code Systems. Chapter 5 in *Health Information Management Technology: An Applied Approach*, 6th ed. N. B. Sayles and L. Gordon, eds. Chicago: AHIMA.

Giannangelo, K. 2019. *Healthcare Code Sets, Clinical Terminologies, and Classification Systems*, 4th ed. Chicago: AHIMA.

1.18 Interoperability

Competency I.6

Read the Office of the National Coordinator for Healthcare Information Technology's paper "Connecting Health and Care for the Nation: A Ten-Year Vision to Achieve Interoperable Health IT Infrastructure." Within the paper, the ONC presents five building blocks for interoperability. Give your opinion on which one will be the most challenging, and provide support for your position.

Resource

Office of the National Coordinator for Health Information Technology. 2016. Connecting Health and Care for the Nation: A Ten-Year Vision to Achieve Interoperable Health IT Infrastructure. https://www.healthit.gov/sites/default/files/ONC10yearInteroperabilityConceptPaper.pdf.

1.19 Information governance advocacy

Competency I.2

1. Two months ago, as HIM director, you broach the subject of information governance (IG) with your immediate boss, the chief financial officer, stating that the formation of a new committee dedicated to IG would be advantageous. Appraise the value of an IG committee and plan for your boss.

2. At the time, the CFO gave you little support for the endeavor. However, today, you hear from your counterpart in IT that she was asked last week to serve on a new committee for information governance that will have its first meeting in two days. You decide to schedule a meeting with the CFO to defend the value that an HIM representative could bring to an IG committee by compiling a comparison of the IG Principles of Healthcare to the responsibilities that HIM already upholds. Use that information to justify your position to add HIM to the IG committee.

Resources

AHIMA. 2019. Information Governance Toolkit 3.0. https://bok.ahima.org/PdfView?oid=302242.

AHIMA. 2016. Information Governance: Principles for Healthcare. http://www.ahima.org/topics/ infogovernance/igbasics?tabid=overview.

1.20 Encoder replacement

Competency I.2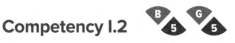

As the coding supervisor for a mid-size acute care hospital, you have been hearing complaints about the current encoder product for the past year. The present contract with the encoder vendor you now have expires in one year. You have received approval to investigate an encoder change.

Construct a timeline for the entire process and assume that you *will* change to a new vendor. Incorporate the steps of the systems development life cycle in your plan.

Resource

Amatayakul, M. K. 2020. Health Information Systems Strategic Planning. Chapter 13 in *Health Information Management Concepts, Principles, and Practice*, 6th ed. P. Oachs and A. Watters, eds. Chicago: AHIMA.

1.21 Screen design for enterprise master patient index

Competency I.2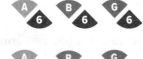

Competency I.6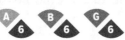

Experiment with building a screen design. Choose the data elements that you would want in an enterprise master patient index (eMPI) and then build a layout of those data elements.

Resources

Reynolds, R. B. and A. Morey. 2020. Health Record Content and Documentation. Chapter 4 in *Health Information Management: Concepts, Principles, and Practice*, 6th ed. P. Oachs and A. Watters, eds. Chicago: AHIMA.

Sayles, N. B. 2020. Health Information Functions, Purpose, and Users. Chapter 3 in *Health Information Management Technology: An Applied Approach*, 6th ed. N. B. Sayles. and L. Gordon, eds. Chicago: AHIMA.

1.22 Cloud computing pros and cons

Competency I.2

The IT director has asked for a meeting with you to discuss the possibility of utilizing cloud computing.

1. Prepare for the meeting by researching cloud computing in healthcare and creating a list of at least three pros and three cons related to the implementation or use of cloud computing. Focus on areas such as cost, access, privacy and security, and performance.

2. Reach a recommendation to share with the IT director at the meeting justifying your position on whether or not implementing cloud computing is a sound practice.

Resources

Amatayakul, M. K. 2020. Health Information Systems Strategic Planning. Chapter 13 in *Health Information Management Concepts, Principles, and Practice*, 6th ed. P. Oachs and A. Watters, eds. Chicago: AHIMA.

Dinh, A. K. 2011. Cloud computing 101. *Journal of AHIMA* 82(4):36–37.

1.23 SNOMED CT versus ICD-10

Competency I.5

Your fellow classmate is having difficulty understanding the difference between SNOMED-CT and ICD-10. Compare the terminologies and distinguish reasons for their usage to assist your classmate with comprehending these concepts.

B

Resources

Bowman, S. 2005. Coordinating SNOMED-CT and ICD-10: Getting the Most out of Electronic Health Record Systems. *Journal of AHIMA* 76(7):60–61.

Palkie, B. 2020. Clinical Classifications, Vocabularies, Terminologies, and Standards. Chapter 5 in *Health Information Management Concepts, Principles, and Practice*, 6th ed. P. Oachs and A. Watters, eds. Chicago: AHIMA.

1.24 Patient registration impact on HIM

Competency I.1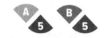

On your first day as HIM director at a small community hospital, your coding staff has come to you complaining about the number of errors originating from patient registration. Over the course of the next week, you see how these errors are impacting the entire revenue cycle from duplicate medical record numbers to wrong insurances listed.

1. Assess the possible reasons for the errors.

2. Present the need and plan for reducing the number of errors to the patient registration director.

Resources

Amatayakul, M. K. 2020. Health Information Systems. Chapter 11 in *Health Information Management Technology: An Applied Approach*, 6th ed. N. B. Sayles and L. Gordon, eds. Chicago: AHIMA.

Cummins, R. and J. Waddell. 2005. Coding Connections in Revenue Cycle Management. *Journal of AHIMA* 76(7):72–74.

Reynolds, R. B. and A. Morey. 2020. Health Record Content and Documentation. Chapter 4 in *Health Information Management: Concepts, Principles, and Practice*, 6th ed. P. Oachs and A. Watters, eds. Chicago: AHIMA.

1.25 Research interoperability

Competency I.6

A research team approaches you, the director of information technology, to determine if there is a way to integrate data from the organization's EHR into their study documents housed in a different vendor platform.

1. Theorize why fulfilling this request would be beneficial to the research team.

2. Suppose you agree to facilitate this project. You surmise the continuity of care document would support interoperability between the two systems. What makes it a good choice?

3. Predict at least three problems that may arise surrounding interoperability.

Resources

Amatayakul, M. K. 2020. Health Information Systems. Chapter 11 in *Health Information Management Technology: An Applied Approach*, 6th ed. N. B. Sayles and L. Gordon, eds. Chicago: AHIMA.

Laird-Maddox, M., S. B. Mitchell, and M. Hoffman. 2014. "Integrating Research Data Capture into the Electronic Health Record Workflow: Real-World Experience to Advance Innovation." *Perspectives in Health Information Management*, Fall 2014. http://perspectives.ahima.org/integrating-research-data -capture-into-the-electronic-health-record-workflow-real-world-experience-to-advance-innovation/.

1.26 Data dictionary and the Joint Commission

Competency I.6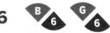

A new hospital is preparing to open. They want to ensure that, when it is time to report on the national quality measures to the Joint Commission, the data flows properly.

1. Assist in creating the data dictionary for the following data elements to be reported by noting the correct format and allowable values.

2. Identify and use the appropriate source document for the quality measures.
   - Admission date
   - Discharge disposition
   - Sex
   - Race
   - Hispanic ethnicity
   - Payment source

Resource

Joint Commission on Accreditation of Healthcare Organizations (Joint Commission). 2019. Specifications Manual for Joint Commission National Quality Measures. https://www .jointcommission.org/specifications_manual_joint_commission_national_quality_core_measures .aspx.

1.27 Data dictionary maintenance

Competency I.5DM

Competency I.6

Currently, in your organization, pediatric patients are considered those that are under 13 years of age. Patients that are admitted to the pediatric unit are registered as PEDS. Reports to your state pediatric disease registry are run based on the location of PEDS. Suppose the state's data dictionary for the pediatric disease registry supplies the definition of pediatric patient as one that is 18 years of age or younger.

1. How will you design or modify reports based on the current data dictionary?

2. Elaborate on what changes need to be made going forward to collect the appropriate information for reporting.

Resources

Brinda, D. 2020. Data Management. Chapter 6 in *Health Information Management Technology: An Applied Approach*, 6th ed. N. B. Sayles and L. Gordon, eds. Chicago: AHIMA.

Davoudi, S., J. Flanigan, S. Houser, L. Kadlec, A. Kirby, D. VanSlyke, and A. Wendicke. 2016. Managing a data dictionary. http://library.ahima.org/PB/DataDictionary.

A

B

G

1.28 Data dictionary flaw

A

B

G

Competency I.6DM

Competency I.6

It has been discovered that there are issues with reporting your organization's Joint Commission core measures because several data elements are incorrectly formatted. You must review the following data elements to isolate the problems and provide the appropriate modification to correct your data submission.

Data element	Current depiction	Revision needed	Correction
Admission date	MM-DD-YY		
Discharge disposition	1-8		
Sex	0, 1, 2		
Race	1-7		
Hispanic	1, 2		
Payment Source	1-12		

Resources

Brinda, D. 2020. Data Management. Chapter 6 in *Health Information Management Technology: An Applied Approach*, 6th ed. N. B. Sayles and L. Gordon, eds. Chicago: AHIMA.

Joint Commission on Accreditation of Healthcare Organizations (Joint Commission). 2019. Specifications Manual for Joint Commission National Quality Measures (v2018A1). https://www.jointcommission.org/specifications_manual_joint_commission_national_quality_core_measures.aspx.

1.29 Data dictionary mapping

Competency I.6DM

Competency I.6

Create a table to map the data element "patient race" to Joint Commission, MEDPAR, and HL7 data requirements. Your organization lists eight race choices and uses the first two letters of each race as the data value.

Patient Race	Facility Code	HL7	MEDPAR	Joint Commission
White	WH			
Black	BL			
Asian	AS			
Native American	NA			
Hispanic	HI			
Pacific Islander	PA			
Other	OT			
Unable to determine	UN			

Resources

AHIMA. 2012. Managing a data dictionary. *Journal of AHIMA* 83(1):48–52.

AHIMA. 2011. Data mapping best practices. *Journal of AHIMA* 82(4):46–52.

HL7. 2019. Appendix A. Data Definition Tables. https://www.hl7.org/special/committees/vocab/V26 _Appendix_A.pdf.

Joint Commission on Accreditation of Healthcare Organizations (Joint Commission). 2019. Specifications Manual for Joint Commission National Quality Measures (v2018A1). https://www .jointcommission.org/specifications_manual_joint_commission_national_quality_core_measures .aspx.

Research Data Distribution Center Medicare Provider Analysis and Review (MEDPAR) Record. 2019. Dictionary for SAS and CSV Datasets. https://www.cms.gov/Research-Statistics-Data-and-Systems /Files-for-Order/IdentifiableDataFiles/Downloads/sasIDmedpar.pdf.

1.30 Evolving leadership roles in HIM

Competency I.1

1. Increased adoption of health information technology is opening innovative leadership pathways for HIM professionals. Four areas of opportunity based on the HIT roadmap created by the Office of the National Coordinator for Health Information Technology include privacy and security, adoption of information technology, interoperability, and collaborative governance. Choose one of these to explore and determine the challenges and opportunities for HIM professionals.

2. Leverage the 3 I's Leadership Model for e-HIM that AHIMA adapted to address one of those challenges.

3. Justify how earning an AHIMA credential can prepare you for leadership opportunity.

Resources

AHIMA. 2016a. e-HIM Overview and Instructions. AHIMA Leadership Model. http://library.ahima.org /xpedio/groups/public/documents/ahima/bok1_042565.pdf.

AHIMA. 2016b. Why Get Certified. Certification. http://www.ahima.org/certification/whycertify.

Dimick, C. 2012. Health information management 2025: Current "health IT revolution" drastically changes HIM in the near future. *Journal of AHIMA* 83(8): 24–31.

1.31 HIM leadership roles

Competency I.1

1. Create an organizational chart for this HIM department.

2. Identify the leadership positions within the department and provide a brief summary of the responsibilities for each leadership role.
   - Melissa Reynolds: Coding supervisor
   - Janet Jefferson: Transcriptionist
   - Margie Brown: Transcriptionist
   - Lois Evers: HIM director
   - Mildred Cabot: Coder
   - Herman Goddard: Assistant HIM director
   - Karen Marshall: Coder
   - Edna George: Lead coder
   - Shirley Richards: Transcription supervisor
   - Taylor Smith: ROI clerk
   - Carol Fredrickson: Scanner tech
   - Josh Maynor: Scanner tech
   - Lisa Hubbard: Coder
   - Gloria Lawson: Transcriptionist
   - Denise Cavanaugh: Coder
   - Laura Benson: ROI clerk
   - Delores Miles: Analyst
   - Kathy Jones: HIM department supervisor
   - Joyce Call: Analyst
   - Carla Wilson: Transcriptionist
   - Leah Carson: Coder
   - Beth McMahon: Analyst
   - Rebecca Morris: Lead transcriptionist

Resource

Sayles, N. B. 2020. Health Information Functions, Purpose, and Users. Chapter 3 in *Health Information Management Technology: An Applied Approach*, 6th ed. N. B. Sayles and L. Gordon, eds. Chicago: AHIMA.

1.32 Institute of Medicine impact

Competency I.1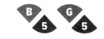

Provide an interpretation of at least four drivers of clinical quality that the Institute of Medicine's reports: *To Err is Human: Building a Safer Health System* and *Crossing the Quality Chasm: A New Health System for the 21st Century* fostered for patient safety (Kohn et al. 2000).

Reference

Kohn, L. T., J. M. Corrigan, and M. S. Donaldson, eds. 2000. *To Err is Human: Building a Safer Health System.* https://www.ncbi.nlm.nih.gov/books/NBK225182/toc/?report=reader.

Resources

Carter, D. and M. N. Palmer. 2020. Performance Improvement. Chapter 18 in *Health Information Management Technology: An Applied Approach*, 6th ed. N. B. Sayles and L. Gordon, eds. Chicago: AHIMA.

O'Dell, R. 2020. Clinical Quality Management. Chapter 20 in *Health Information Management: Concepts, Principles, and Practice*, 6th ed. P. Oachs and A. Watters, eds. Chicago: AHIMA.

1.33 Accountable care organization, information governance, and strategic planning

Competency I.1

You have taken the HIM director position for an accountable care organization (ACO). One of the first areas you have been tasked to focus on is incorporation of information governance (IG) into the organization. The CEO has indicated that most administrative staff see IG as solely an HIM strategy, which deals with proper release of information and record retention or destruction. Your first recommendation is the creation of an IG team or council where you can ensure that the stakeholders understand the value of IG to the ACO and can then work together to assure compliance.

Another area of focus is the development of a new HIM strategic plan. The old strategic plan was centered around customer service (release of information) and reimbursement. Your plan is to revise the plan to include goals that include IG and ACOs.

The third area that you decide should be addressed relates to registries. While the individual organizations within the ACO report to such registries as the state trauma registry or the national or state cancer registries, creation of patient registries within the ACO could be a valuable tool. This will require the support of the CEO as additional staffing will need to be hired to create and maintain the registries.

1. Evaluate the relationship of information governance (IG) to ACOs.

2. Which organizational stakeholders would you recommend be on the IG team/council for an ACO?

3. The HIM department's strategic plan needs revised to include IG and ACOs. What goals would you include for those strategies?

4. Justify the use of registries in facilitating an accountable care organization's strategies.

Resources

Acker, B. M., P. Bankowski-Petz, and S. Costello, et al. 2017. Information Governance Toolkit 3.0. http://bok.ahima.org/PdfView?oid=302242.

McClernon, S. E. 2020. Strategic Thinking and Management. Chapter 28 in *Health Information Management: Concepts, Principles, and Practice*, 6th ed. P. Oachs and A. Watters, eds. Chicago: AHIMA.

Viola, A. and L. Washington. 2011. Accountable Care: Implications for Managing Health Information. AHIMA Thought Leadership Series. http://library.ahima.org/xpedio/groups/public/documents/ahima/bok1_049111.pdf.

Washington, L. 2015. Information Governance Offers a Strategic Approach for Healthcare. *Journal of AHIMA* 86(11):56–59.

White, S., C. Kallem, A. Viola, and J. Bronnert. 2011. An ACO primer: Reviewing the proposed rule on accountable care organizations. *Journal of AHIMA* 82(6):48–50.

1.34 Information governance plan

Competency I.2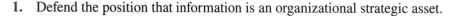

1. Defend the position that information is an organizational strategic asset.

2. Explain the importance of having an information governance plan in place to manage an organization's information assets.

Resource

Fahy, K., C. Leonhard, N. Miller, and J. Wiens. 2018. Information Governance Offers a Strategic Approach for Healthcare. http://bok.ahima.org/doc?oid=302617#.XQwat49OmUk.

1.35 Data dictionary

Competency I.6

1. A data dictionary for patient address and phone number is shown below. Margaret, a registration clerk, is trying to enter the patient's state of Arizona. Every time she starts typing it, Arkansas pops up. Identify the issue preventing the correct state from being entered.

2. Margaret begins to enter the patient's telephone number of 616-256-6767 and only gets as far as 616-256-67 and the field will not accept any more characters. Identify this issue and how it can be corrected.

Field Name	Data Type	Description
Patient_Street	Text	Street address
Patient_City	Text	City name
Patient_State	Text	Postal code for the state
Patient_Zip code	Text	5 digit zip code
Patient_Phone	Text	Phone number

Resources

Brinda, D. 2020. Data Management. Chapter 6 in *Health Information Management Technology: An Applied Approach*, 6th ed. N. B. Sayles and L. Gordon, eds. Chicago: AHIMA.

Sharp, M. and C. Madlock-Brown. 2020. Data Management. Chapter 6 in *Health Information Management: Concepts, Principles, and Practice*, 6th ed. P. Oachs and A. Watters, eds. Chicago: AHIMA.

1.36 Managed care versus accountable care

Competency I.1

Competency I.1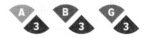

You are the office manager for an orthopedic surgeon who consistently meets annual quality benchmarks. He has a strong relationship with the hospital where he has privileges and uses the hospital's information system efficiently, as evidenced by the lack of duplicative services, such as MRIs or CT scans.

The surgeon is trying to decide whether to join an accountable care organization (ACO) or stay under the managed care organization he has been with for the past several years. He approaches you for clarity.

a. Provide a comparison of the two organizations for the surgeon, noting their characteristics.

b. Then provide a recommendation for his participation.

Resource

Casto, A. B. 2018. *Principles of Healthcare Reimbursement,* 6th ed. Chicago: AHIMA.

1.37 Data stewardship

Competency I.2

1. Jim has just been hired as a cancer registrar at a large tertiary care facility. He will be one of four abstractors for the registry. After two days of job training spent going over the registry's data dictionary definitions, Jim is frustrated. He wants to dig in and start abstracting actual cases. Educate Jim on the importance of the data dictionary and the correct application of its definitions for the registry.

2. Apply the concept of data stewardship to this process.

Resources

Brinda, D. 2020. Data Management. Chapter 6 in *Health Information Management Technology: An Applied Approach*, 6th ed. N. B. Sayles and L. Gordon, eds. Chicago: AHIMA.

Johns, M. 2020. Data Governance and Stewardship. Chapter 3 in *Health Information Management Concepts, Principles, and Practice*, 6th ed. P. Oachs and A. Watters, eds. Chicago: AHIMA.

Sharp, M. 2020. Secondary Data Sources. Chapter 7 in *Health Information Management Technology: An Applied Approach*, 6th ed. N. B. Sayles and L. Gordon, eds. Chicago: AHIMA.

1.38 Data quality management

Competency I.2

A new EHR is going to be purchased for the physician practice you manage. Use three of the characteristics of data quality from AHIMA's Data Quality Management Model and illustrate how incorporating those characteristics into the EHR will support patient care decisions.

Resources

Brinda, D. 2020. Data Management. Chapter 6 in *Health Information Management Technology: An Applied Approach*, 6th ed. N. B. Sayles and L. Gordon, eds. Chicago: AHIMA.

Davoudi, S., J. A. Dooling, B. Glondys, et al. 2015. Data Quality Management Model. *Journal of AHIMA* 86(10): expanded web version.

1.39 Information management plan

Competency I.2

Your organization's strategic plan incorporates the following tenets:

- Excel in quality patient care
- Provide exceptional service
- Enhance the patient care environment and facility infrastructure
- Foster partnership
  - Internally: staff, physicians, leadership
  - Externally: community
- Maintain financial stability through efficiency and growth

The information management plan needs to be updated to espouse those principles. Determine an objective that would fit each of these tenets to incorporate in the information management plan and supply the rationale(s) for each objective's inclusion.

Resource

Gordon, L. 2020. Management. Chapter 17 in *Health Information Management Technology: An Applied Approach*, 6th ed. N. B. Sayles and L. Gordon, eds. Chicago: AHIMA.

1.40 HIM department strategic plan

Competency I.2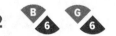

Your organization's strategic plan incorporates the following tenets:
- Excel in quality patient care
- Provide exceptional service
- Enhance the patient care environment and facility infrastructure
- Foster partnership
  - Internally: staff, physicians, leadership
  - Externally: community
- Maintain financial stability through efficiency and growth

Create an HIM mission and vision statement that promotes those principles.

Resources

Gordon, L. 2020. Management. Chapter 17 in *Health Information Management Technology: An Applied Approach,* 6th ed. N. B. Sayles and L. Gordon, eds. Chicago: AHIMA.

O'Dell, R. M. 2020. Clinical Quality Management. Chapter 20 in *Health Information Management: Concepts, Principles, and Practice*, 6th ed. P. Oachs and A. Watters, eds. Chicago: AHIMA.

1.41 Password management

Competency I.3

At Pine Valley Community Hospital (PVCH), passwords are required to be a minimum of five characters and must contain one number. HIM clerk Julie was hired more than a year ago and has yet to be prompted to change her password. This gave her concern, as she recalled password management best practices from her recent studies.

1. What recommendations might Julie make to improve password management at PVCH?

2. Create an example of a secure password and justify the selection.

3. Determine if the password #SnU75* would meet the requirements you provided and justify your response.

Resource

Sayles, N. B. and L. Kavanaugh-Burke. 2018. *Introduction to Information Systems for Health Information Technology*, 3rd ed. Chicago: AHIMA.

1.42 Data quality model

Competency I.3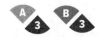

Conduct an internet search to find AHIMA's Data Quality Model. Select which characteristic of data from the model is factoring into the scenarios below.

1. The Joint Commission states that patient discharge time should be noted in hours (00–23) and minutes (00–59) or as UTD (unable to determine). Your information system was set up to capture discharge time in hours (00–12), minutes (00–59), and AM or PM.

2. During abstracting, an HIM clerk identifies that the results of an MRI were never dictated.

3. The radiology director is reviewing the 2020 CPT code changes today (1/31/2020) that affect her chargemaster. She will send a list of updates to the chargemaster committee for implementation next week.

4. Gretchen is attempting to code a prostatectomy for patient Gerry Jefferies. When she enters the CPT code the system will not take it. She tries again, knowing she has the correct code and the system still will not accept the code. Then she looks at the patient's sex listed in the system and finds it is female.

Resource

Sayles, N. B. and L. Kavanaugh-Burke. 2018. *Introduction to Information Systems for Health Information Technology*, 3rd ed. Chicago: AHIMA.

1.43 Data integrity

Competency I.3

1. In your current electronic health record (EHR), registration clerks often bypass the admitting diagnosis field. This is a problem because coders work from a list that pulls the information to be coded. What initiative can you request with your next update to eliminate that problem?

2. If you implement the initiative you identified, will the problem be totally eliminated? Explain your answer.

Resource

Sayles, N. B. and L. Kavanaugh-Burke. 2018. *Introduction to Information Systems for Health Information Technology*, 3rd ed. Chicago: AHIMA.

1.44 Intrusion detection

Competency I.3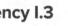

As the information technology manager for a large physician practice, you are concerned about unauthorized system access. You want to invest in an intrusion detection system (IDS) to monitor the IT system in real-time. Defend this choice to the practice physicians who are reluctant to invest in an IDS.

Resource

Rinehart-Thompson, L. 2018. *Introduction to Health Information Privacy and Security*, 2nd ed. Chicago: AHIMA.

1.45 Corrections

Competency I.3

You are the coding manager for a large city hospital. You outsource some overflow coding to a vendor. As the contact person for those coders, you sometimes get emails asking for discharge dates or dispositions to be entered so the account can be finalized. You would like those coders to be able to enter that information themselves to save you time. Your HIM director has a differing opinion. What explanations would lead you to support her position?

Resource

Sayles, N. B. 2020. Health Information Functions, Purposes, and Users. Chapter 3 in *Health Information Management Technology: An Applied Approach*, 6th ed. N. B. Sayles and L. Gordon, eds. Chicago: AHIMA.

A

B

1.46 Telemedicine I

Competency I.1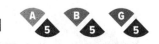

Eve Lawrence, the HIM director at Willow Falls, a critical access hospital in southeastern Ohio, first heard about the new teleradiology program the hospital wants to implement at a department head meeting today. The CEO stated that he already vetted several different radiology groups that might provide this teleradiology service, which the board of directors would like to have in place next month. He narrowed the selection down to these three: Johnson Radiology Associates, Nationwide Radiology Group, and Baskin & Singer Teleradiology Services. The full board will determine which group to use at their next meeting in one week.

Eve wants to be sure that there are no unpleasant surprises with the implementation of this process, so she does research and discovers the following information:

- Johnson Radiology Associates is based in Virginia; all providers are licensed in Virginia; it serves five organizations
- Nationwide Radiology Group is based in Florida; its providers are licensed in Florida, Texas, California, Nevada, Arizona, and New Mexico; it serves 23 organizations
- Baskin & Singer Teleradiology Services is based in Missouri; all providers are licensed in Missouri; in addition, some providers also have licenses in Oklahoma, Texas, Louisiana, Illinois, and Tennessee; it serves 12 organizations

Based on this information, what recommendation should Eve make to the CEO and why?

Resource

Anderson, R., B. Beckett, K. Fahy, et al. 2017. Telemedicine Toolkit. http://bok.ahima.org /PdfView?oid=302358.

1.47 Telemedicine II

Competency I.2

Refer to information presented in scenario 1.46 to complete this exercise.

Eve has additional concerns from an HIM perspective regarding the proposed telemedicine program, which she feels is being rushed into. Justify Eve's concerns by compiling the HIM-related tasks that would need to be addressed prior to implementation of any telemedicine program.

Resource

Anderson, R., B. Beckett, K. Fahy, et al. 2017. Telemedicine Toolkit. http://bok.ahima.org /PdfView?oid=302358.

Johnson, M. L. and D. Warner. 2013. Telemedicine Services and the Health Record (2013 update). http://bok.ahima.org/doc?oid=300269.

1.48 Telemedicine III

Competency I.1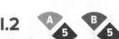

Competency I.2

Refer to information presented in scenarios 1.46 and 1.47 to complete this exercise.

The medical staff secretary, Vanessa, approached Eve after the department meeting with concerns about physician credentialing for telemedicine services. They meet and decide that they must see if there are CMS or Joint Commission rules related to credentialing of telemedicine providers to ensure their critical access facility is in compliance. Determine the credentialing required for telemedicine providers who provide services at Willow Falls.

Resources

Johnson, M. L. and D. Warner. 2013. Telemedicine Services and the Health Record (2013 update). http://bok.ahima.org/doc?oid=300269.

Joint Commission on Accreditation of Healthcare Organizations. 2012. Final Revisions to Telemedicine Standards. Retrieved from https://www.jointcommission.org/assets/1/6 /Revisions_telemedicine_standards.pdf.

Chapter 2

Domain II: Information Protection: Access, Use, Disclosure, Privacy and Security

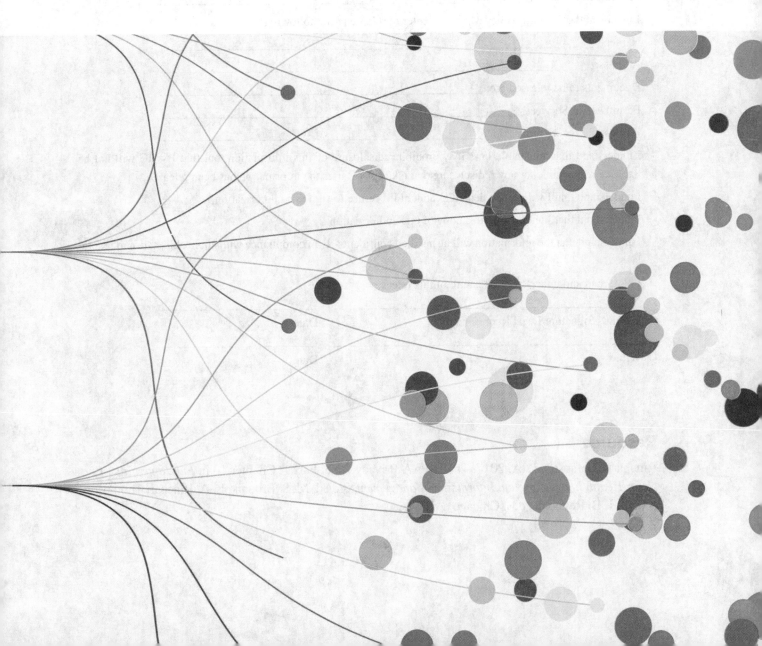

2.0 Release of information form

Competency II.1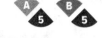

Competency II.3

Assess the following authorization form against the Privacy Rule criteria and determine if any element(s) is(are) missing. Modify the document by adding language to incorporate any element(s) found missing.

PINE VALLEY COMMUNITY HOSPITAL
AUTHORIZATION TO RELEASE HEALTH INFORMATION

Patient's Name: _____ Date of Birth: _____

Patient's Social Security Number: _____

I hereby authorize Pine Valley Medical Center to release to the following:

Name: _____

Address: _____

Documents to be released are: _____

From Date of Service: _____

Purpose for record request is: _____

I understand that applicable laws may prohibit redisclosure of this information, but that PVMC will not be liable or responsible for any redisclosure that takes place after the information has been released.

I understand that I will not be denied treatment if I refuse to sign this authorization.

I understand that I am entitled to a copy of this authorization.

I understand that the information will be handled confidentially in compliance with applicable state and federal laws.

I have read and understand the nature of this release.

_____   _____
Patient's Signature/Legal Representative   Date

_____   _____
Witness   Date

Resource

Rinehart-Thompson, L. A. 2017. The HIPAA Privacy Rule: Part 1. Chapter 10 in *Fundamentals of Law for Health Informatics and Information Management,* 3rd ed. M. S. Brodnik, L. A. Rinehart-Thompson, and R. B. Reynolds, eds. Chicago: AHIMA.

2.1 Security policy—HIM student practicum

Competency II.1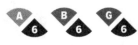

Competency II.2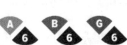

Your HIM department is going to begin taking students as part of their Professional Practice Experience (PPE). The HIM director has asked you to create a short educational program on privacy, security, and confidentiality for the students to complete before they start their PPE. Create a PowerPoint presentation of no more than 12 slides that covers the following elements:

- Differentiate between privacy, security, and confidentiality
- Access to be based on minimum necessary standard
- Release of information requires authorization
- Use and protection of passwords and security codes
- Duty to report breaches

Resources

AHIMA. n.d. Professional Practice Experience Guide Version V. Accessed 21 June 2019.https://www. ahima.org/ppe.

Miaoulis, W. M. 2014. Information Security—An Overview (2014 update). http://library.ahima.org/PB /InformationSecurity#.XETuNVVKi70.

2.2 Information access

Competency II.1

Analyze the following scenarios to determine who can appropriately access health information.

1. Mrs. John Smith is requesting the emergency department records from last week of her daughter, Katy. Mrs. Smith is the noncustodial parent of Katy, who lives with her dad. Should you release the records to her? Why or why not?

2. Mr. Fred Mitchell is requesting the birth record for Amy, his birth daughter. Mr. and Mrs. Mitchell gave Amy up for adoption four years ago. Should you release the records to him? Why or why not?

3. Mrs. Lynn Olsen is requesting the lab results of her husband, Tim. She has a note, signed by him, giving his permission for her to have the records. Should you release the records to her? Why or why not?

4. An investigator from Homeland Security is requesting patient records as part of an ongoing investigation. Should you release the information to the investigator? Why or why not?

5. Dr. Rex Harrison is requesting the medical records of Martha Flynn. He states he is a family friend and has been asked by Mrs. Flynn's son to review her last inpatient admission for appropriateness of care. Should you release the records to Dr. Harrison? Why or why not?

Resource

Brodnik, M. S. 2017. Access, Use, and Disclosure and Release of Health Information. Chapter 15 in *Fundamentals of Law for Health Informatics and Information Management,* 3rd ed. M. S. Brodnik, L. A. Rinehart-Thompson, and R. B. Reynolds, eds. Chicago: AHIMA.

2.3 Potential privacy violation

Competency II.2

On 11/23/19, the mayor of your town was seen in your emergency department and subsequently admitted with injuries that included an orbital floor blow-out fracture and multiple bruises until discharge on the 26th. Past rumors have hinted that the mayor is in an abusive relationship and speculation is rampant that these injuries are a result of abuse. Since the incident, local newspapers have printed health information that should not be available to them. To address a potential privacy breach, the IT department ran an audit trail to see who had accessed the patient's records. Five employees in the HIM department accessed the record, and you are tasked with determining if any of them violated the privacy policy.

At this facility, records are still hybrid.

The employees are:
  N. Northwest, coder
  L. Easton, coder
  S. Southward, transcriptionist
  E. Downey, file clerk
  W. Upton, file clerk

Following is the audit trail you were given from IT.

Audit Trail for MR#655966	
User	**Date**
N. Northwest	11/28/2019
S. Southward	11/27/2019
L. Easton	11/26/2019
E. Downey	11/24/2019
W. Upton	11/29/2019

What other relevant elements will you ask IT to include in the audit trail?

Resources

Rinehart-Thompson, L. A. 2018. HIPAA Security Rule Concepts. Chapter 4 in *Introduction to Health Information Privacy and Security*, 2nd ed. Chicago: AHIMA.

Walsh, T. and W. M. Miaoulis, 2014. Practice Brief: Privacy and security audits of electronic health information. *Journal of AHIMA* 85(3): 54–59.

2.4 HIM staff privacy and security education

Competency II.1

Competency II.2

You want to provide ongoing privacy and security training for your 25 HIM staff. The HIM department is diverse: workers range in age from 25–62; three men; four Latinos, two African-Americans, and the remainder Caucasian; four of your older staff still struggle with computer literacy; 11 are college graduates (seven baccalaureate degrees, four associate degrees); one staff member is in a wheelchair; and 12 work from home.

1. From this information, theorize at least three delivery methods that might be considered in order to have successful privacy and security education.

2. Identify at least five cultural or diversity issues that could raise barriers during the training.

3. Formulate a plan for educating your HIM staff on privacy and security. (The focus of this portion of the assignment is not the content of the education but the delivery method[s] to be used.)

Resources

AHIMA. 2003. Think salad, not stew: managing cultural differences in your HIM department. *AHIMA Advantage* 7:1.

Hamilton, M. 2020. Ethical Issues in Health Information Management. Chapter 21 in *Health Information Management Technology: An Applied Approach*, 6th ed. N. Sayles and L. Gordon, eds. Chicago: AHIMA.

Patena, K. 2020. Employee Training and Development. Chapter 23 in *Health Information Management: Concepts, Principles, and Practice*, 6th ed. P. Oachs and A. Watters, eds. Chicago: AHIMA.

Prater, V. S. 2020. Human Resources Management and Professional Development. Chapter 20 in *Health Information Management Technology: An Applied Approach*, 6th ed. N. Sayles and L. Gordon, eds. Chicago: AHIMA.

2.5 Privacy and security education

Competency II.1

Competency II.2

As the HIM director at Pine Valley Community Hospital, a critical access hospital, you are also the privacy and security officer for the organization. You are preparing an annual privacy and security training for nonclinical staff.

Create a slide presentation (minimum of 20 slides) to be provided at an in-service along with a short post-test (10 questions). Make sure to cover the relevant HIPAA and HITECH information for these nonclinical staff, including a distinction between privacy, security, and confidentiality.

Resource

AHIMA. 2014. Practice Brief: Information security—an overview. http://bok.ahima.org
    /doc?oid=300244#.XRfnhutKi70.

2.6 HIM department breach

Competency II.1

Competency II.2

On 10/14/18, a well-known local politician died in your emergency department from injuries sustained in a motor vehicle accident. The record was entered in the EHR on the 14th, additional documents scanned on the 15th, and the record was coded on the 16th.

As part of the normal course of business, the IT department ran an audit trail to see who had accessed the patient's records. Five employees in the HIM department accessed the record, and you are tasked with determining if any of them violated privacy policy.
(At this facility, records are still hybrid.)

The employees are:

N. Northwest—coder

L. Easton—coder

S. Southward—transcriptionist

E. Downey—file clerk

W. Upton—file clerk

1. Based on the audit trail below, formulate an opinion on whether or not any of these employees may have violated the privacy policy. Support your decision.

Audit Trail for MR#655966				
User	**Date**	**Workstation**	**Application Accessed**	**Action**
N. Northwest	10/16/2018	Home workstation 12	EHR, encoder, lab, radiology	R, M, R, R
S. Southward	10/15/2018	Home workstation 18	EHR, transcription system, radiology	R, M, M
L. Easton	10/17/2018	Home workstation 9	EHR, lab, radiology	R, R, R
E. Downey	10/15/2018	8th floor nurse's station	EHR, lab, radiology	R, R, R
W. Upton	10/15/2018	HIM department workstation 3	EHR, Chart tracking system	R, M
R = Read				
M = Modified				

2. Propose the next steps to take if there was a concern that one or more the employees violated the privacy policy.

Resource

Rinehart-Thompson, L. A. 2018. HIPAA Security Rule Concepts. Chapter 4 in *Introduction to Health Information Privacy and Security*, 2nd ed. Chicago: AHIMA.

Walsh, T. and W. M. Miaoulis. 2014. Practice Brief: Privacy and security audits of electronic health information. *Journal of AHIMA* 85(3): 54–59.

2.7 Back-ups and e-discovery

Competency II.3

You are the recently hired health information manager for a very large physician group practice. You are reviewing policies and procedures related to e-discovery and notice that there is no mention of a policy related to back-up media. You contact the information technology manager who says that she tried to address this issue a year ago, but the practice group manager did not feel it was important, stating it was covered under HIM policies related to retention and destruction. You decide to hold a meeting to reintroduce the topic.

1. Determine who should take part in the meeting.

2. Assume that you will get pushback for addressing this topic again. Offer insight to the group on why this topic must be addressed.

Resources

Baldwin-Stried Reich, K. and K. Downing. 2013. E- Discovery litigation and regulatory investigation response planning: crucial components of your organization's information and data governance processes. *Journal of AHIMA* 84(11): expanded web version.

Klaver, J. C. 2017. Evidence. Chapter 5 in *Fundamentals of Law for Health Informatics and Information Management*, 3rd ed. M. S. Brodnik, L. A. Rinehart, R. B. Reynolds, eds. Chicago: AHIMA.

Rinehart-Thompson, L. A. 2017. Legal Proceedings. Chapter 4 in *Fundamentals of Law for Health Informatics and Information Management*, 3rd ed. M. S. Brodnik, L. A. Rinehart-Thompson, and R. B. Reynolds, eds. Chicago: AHIMA.

2.8 Release of information cost

Competency II.1

Mrs. Smith has requested records from her last inpatient stay in the hospital and states that she will pick the records up when they are ready. Her stay was a result of a motor vehicle accident, and she is requesting the films of her head CT and leg MRI (five films total) be specifically included; additionally, there are 47 total pages that will need to be printed from the EHR. Your state imposes restrictions on what can be charged for production of medical record requests.

1. Using the information below, calculate the cost to Mrs. Smith for her records.
   - For a request made by patients or their representatives, hospitals may charge:
     - $3.40 per page for the first 10 pages,
     - 68 cents per page for pages 11 through 50,
     - 30 cents per page for pages numbering more than 50.
     - With respect to data resulting from an x-ray, MRI, or CAT scan, recorded on paper or film:
       - $3.15 per film
     - The actual cost of postage may be charged.
   - For a request made by someone other than the patient or patient's representative, hospitals may charge:
     - An initial fee of $25.00 to compensate for the records search.
     - $1.75 per page for the first 10 pages,
     - 68 cents per page for pages 11 through 50,
     - 30 cents per page for pages numbering more than 50.
   - With respect to data resulting from an x-ray, MRI, or CAT scan, recorded on paper or film:
     - $3.15 per film
     - The actual cost of postage may be charged.

2. Does the fee change if Mrs. Smith requests an electronic copy of the records?

Resource

Brodnik, M. S. 2017. Access, Use, and Disclosure and Release of Health Information. Chapter 15 in *Fundamentals of Law for Health Informatics and Information Management*, 3rd ed. M. S. Brodnik, L. A. Rinehart-Thompson, R. B. Reynolds, eds. Chicago: AHIMA.

2.9 Release of information error

Competency II.1

Martha, a new release of information clerk is being trained. She has been given a copy of the release of information (ROI) procedure to follow, which is (in part) as follows:

Walk-in requests

1. Validate authorization
2. Process the request
3. Enter the request in the ROI database

On Friday morning, at the end of Martha's first week, a woman stating she was Mrs. Turner walked in requesting her records. Joyce, Martha's trainer, had been called to the HIM director's office, so Martha was on her own. She presented Mrs. Turner with an authorization form, and once it was completed, she printed the records requested. These were lab tests, which included pregnancy results. Martha presented the records to Mrs. Turner, and then proceeded to enter the information into the ROI database as per protocol. When Joyce returned to the office, she reviewed Martha's handling of the request. Joyce became concerned about the request because Mrs. Turner was well known to her and her review of the authorization identified a concern with the signature. When she asked Martha for a description of the woman, her fears were confirmed that it was not Mrs. Turner who had requested the records.

What changes could be recommended to the ROI procedure to ensure that this type of release error would be less likely to happen in the future?

Resource

Brodnik, M. S. 2017. Access, Use, and Disclosure and Release of Health Information. Chapter 15 in *Fundamentals of Law for Health Informatics and Information Management*, 3rd ed. M. S. Brodnik, L. A. Rinehart-Thompson, R. B. Reynolds, eds. Chicago: AHIMA.

2.10 Mobile health technology security

Competency II.1

Competency II.2

Your organization's director of home health services wants to equip her staff with laptops to record patient data. She has done a work study that proves that staff spend a significant amount of time on duplicate work as they collect patient information on paper in the home and then must transfer it into the information system back at the office. The IT director has concerns about the privacy and security of information that would be collected on the laptops. Strategize at least four ways to minimize privacy and security concerns.

Resources

Herzig, T. 2012. Practice Brief: Mobile device security (updated). *Journal of AHIMA* 83(4):50–55.

Miaoulis, W. M. 2014. Practice Brief: Information security—an overview (2014 update). http://bok .ahima.org/doc?oid=300244#.XRfnhutKi70.

Olenik, K. and R. B. Reynolds. 2017. Security Threats and Controls. Chapter 13 in *Fundamentals of Law for Health Informatics and Information Management*, 3rd ed. M. S. Brodnik, L. A. Rinehart-Thompson, and R. B. Reynolds, eds. Chicago: AHIMA.

2.11 Mobile health technology security II

Competency II.1

Competency II.2

Next month, Three River Home Health nursing staff are going to receive laptops to record patient data while at the patient's home. As Three River's privacy and security consultant, you are well aware that stolen laptops often result in a breach of privacy and security. Design a set of at least four standards for off-site laptop use that can prevent theft.

Resources

Herzig, T. 2012. Practice Brief: Mobile device security (updated). *Journal of AHIMA* 83(4):50–55.

Miaoulis, W. M. and T. Walsh. 2014. Practice Brief: Information security—an overview. http://bok .ahima.org/doc?oid=300244#.XRfnhutKi70.

2.12 Disaster recovery planning

Competency II.2

You have been hired as the privacy and security director of a rural community hospital in southern Maine, which has 45 beds. You decide to begin by reviewing the policies and procedures already in place against what is required under HIPAA. You are dismayed to find that although there are a number of policies and procedures in effect, a security risk assessment was never performed. Create a nine-step plan for conducting the security risk assessment.

Resource

Walsh, T. 2013. Practice Brief: Security risk analysis and management: an overview (updated). http://library.ahima.org/doc?oid=300266#.XEeSrlVKi70.

2.13 Security audit

Competency II.1

Competency II.2

Pine Valley Community Hospital just hired a new IT director. She is reviewing recent audit information and notices that audits are only being performed when there is a VIP receiving care. She reaches out to you in your role as HIM director for your opinion on what other circumstances should prompt an audit. Take it a step further and offer suggestions for how often the audits should take place.

Resource

Walsh, T. 2014. Practice Brief: Security audits of electronic health information (updated). *Journal of AHIMA* 85(3):54–59.

2.14 Patient mix-up

Competency II.1

In the group family practice where you are the administrator for six participating physicians, patients share a waiting room. Patients are called by first name to go to their respective physician's exam room. The third patient of the day was Ted Jones, Jr. He sees Dr. Williams, but his father, Ted Jones, Sr. sees Dr. Morrison. When his name is called, he is placed in an exam room for Dr. Morrison. Twenty minutes later, when Dr. Morrison comes in, they realize he was placed in the wrong room. He now has to wait another thirty minutes to see the correct physician and is very irate when he leaves. Later that same day, Karen Smith is registered to see Dr. Cole. She steps out to the restroom and the newly hired medical assistant calls for Karen. Karen Maxwell gets up and goes in for her first visit with Dr. Cole and it is not until the medical assistant asks about her response to the medication that was prescribed at the last visit that they realize the patient is not Karen Smith. You recommend that the practice implement a patient verification policy to prevent these types of errors in the future. What criteria would you include in the policy at registration and in the examination room?

Resource

Dooling, J., S. Durkin, L. Fernandes, B. Just, S. Kotyk, E. Shakespeare Karl, and K. Westhafer. 2014. Managing the integrity of patient identity in health information exchange (2014 update). *Journal of AHIMA* 85(5):60–65.

2.15 E-discovery preservation

Competency II.1

Competency II.2

Competency II.3

As the new privacy officer of St. Stephen's Hospital, you establish an e-discovery committee after learning that several legal cases were settled due to premature record destruction. Several task force members propose that the hospital's attorney notify the privacy officer when litigation has begun so that the e-discovery process can be initiated internally. However, your proposal is to identify situations that may trigger litigation in the first place, so that the organization can be proactive in managing the associated documents. What triggers would you recommend to the task force for inclusion in the e-discovery policy and why?

Resources

AHIMA e-Discovery Task Force. 2008. Litigation Response Planning and Policies for E-Discovery. AHIMA Model E-Discovery Policies: Preservation and Legal Hold for Health Information and Records. *Journal of AHIMA* 79(2): BoK Extras.

Klaver, J. C. 2017. Evidence. Chapter 5 in *Fundamentals of Law for Health Informatics and Information Management,* 3rd ed. M. S. Brodnik, L. A. Rinehart-Thompson, and R. B. Reynolds, eds. Chicago: AHIMA.

2.16 E-discovery sources

Competency II.3

1. Once the e-discovery task force has identified the litigation triggers in 2.15, they move on to assessing the locations where organizational information, including the business record, legal health record, and designated record set, reside in order to include them in the e-discovery policy. Compile a list of at least seven record locations within an organization that should be addressed.

2. The HIM director is a reluctant participant in the task force because he is unsure what skills he brings to the endeavor and presumes this is mostly an IT concern. Persuade him of the value his knowledge base brings to the task force and how that knowledge can influence the e-discovery policy.

Resources

AHIMA e-Discovery Task Force. 2008. Litigation Response Planning and Policies for E-Discovery. AHIMA Model E-Discovery Policies: Preservation and Legal Hold for Health Information and Records. *Journal of AHIMA* 79(2): BoK Extras.

Rinehart-Thompson, L. A. 2020. Legal Issues in Health Information Management. Chapter 2 in *Health Information Management: Concepts, Principles, and Practice*, 6th ed. P. Oachs and A. Watters, eds. Chicago: AHIMA.

2.17 Security access controls

Competency II.2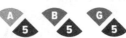

You are the HIM director at a new long-term care facility. You are working with IT to develop access controls for your staff, which will consist of two coders, one scanner tech, one chart analyzer, one clerk who will handle release of information and incomplete records, and three transcriptionists.

1. Analyze the three different types of access controls noting the differences.
2. Recommend which type of access control to assign to each staff member.

Resource

Olenik, K. and R. B. Reynolds. 2017. Security Threats and Controls. Chapter 13 in *Fundamentals of Law for Health Informatics and Information Management,* 3rd ed. M. S. Brodnik, L. A. Rinehart-Thompson, and R. B. Reynolds, eds. Chicago: AHIMA.

2.18 Remote access controls

Competency II.1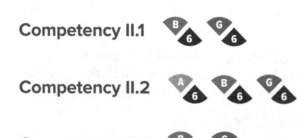

Competency II.2

Competency II.3

As the HIM coding supervisor, you would like to migrate your in-house coding to home-based. In anticipation of concerns that IT might raise about remote access, you have been evaluating best practices for remote security. Your recommendation would be to provide each coder with a laptop for remote access to your organization's information.

1. Elaborate on why this is your choice in view of HIPAA security provisions.

2. Propose at least six other recommendations that would control remote access and promote security.

3. Create a privacy and security policy for remote workers.

Resources

AHIMA Privacy and Security Practice Council. 2007. Safeguards for remote access. *Journal of AHIMA* 78(7):68–70.

Fulmer, K. 2010. Securing remote access to EHRs. *For the Record* 22(18):6.

Miaoulis, W. M. 2014. Practice Brief: Information security—an overview (2014 update). http://bok .ahima.org/doc?oid=300244#.XRfnhutKi70.

Olenik, K. and R. B. Reynolds. 2017. Security Threats and Controls. Chapter 13 in Fundamentals of Law for Health Informatics and Information Management, 3rd ed. M. S. Brodnik, L. A. Rinehart-Thompson, and R. B. Reynolds, eds. Chicago: AHIMA.

2.19 Medical identity theft and personal health records

Competency II.1

Assume that your parents have decided to create individual personal health records (PHRs). They found a vendor, PHRs-R-Us, online and want your advice, as an HIM student, about using their service. They are quick to tell you the vendor is HIPAA-compliant. Differentiate a HIPAA-compliant PHR vendor from one that is offered by a HIPAA-covered entity for your parents and be sure to address your concern about medical identity theft in your response. Recommend a PHR that is provided by a HIPAA-covered entity.

Resources

Rinehart-Thompson, L. A. 2017. Legal Health Record: Maintenance, Content, Documentation, and Disposition. Chapter 9 in *Fundamentals of Law for Health Informatics and Information Management,* 3rd ed. M. S. Brodnik, L. A. Rinehart-Thompson, and R. B. Reynolds, eds. Chicago: AHIMA.

Rinehart-Thompson, L. A. 2008. Raising awareness of medical identity theft: for consumers, prevention starts with guarding, monitoring health information. *Journal of AHIMA* 79(10):74–75, 81.

A

B

2.20 Medical identity theft

A

Competency II.1

Competency II.2

Competency II.3

For each person described in the following scenario, determine if the situation they are involved in is identity theft, medical identity theft, or neither.

Dr. Morehouse is a psychiatrist who employs Daniel as his billing clerk, Laura as his coder, and Kim as his medical assistant. He contracts with Cheryl for janitorial services. As part of his arrangement with Cheryl, she provides him with discarded patient information from other facilities where she works. He then uses the information to submit claims for psychiatric services. Meanwhile, Daniel takes patient account payments by credit card over the phone and uses the credit card numbers and patient information to make online purchases. Laura's unemployed twin sister needs to go to urgent care for treatment for bronchitis. Since she cannot afford the urgent care visit, Laura gives her sister her insurance card so she can get treatment. Kim is a recent hire and still trying to get comfortable with the EHR. Today, while she was entering patient information, she accidently altered the blood type for all patients.

Resources

Olenik, K. and R. B. Reynolds. 2017. Security Threats and Controls. Chapter 13 in *Fundamentals of Law for Health Informatics and Information Management,* 3rd ed. M. S. Brodnik, L. A. Rinehart-Thompson, and R. B. Reynolds, eds. Chicago: AHIMA.

Rinehart-Thompson, L. A. 2008. raising awareness of medical identity theft: for consumers, prevention starts with guarding, monitoring health information. *Journal of AHIMA* 79(10):74–75, 81.

2.21 Confidentiality statement

Competency II.1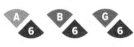

Competency II.2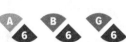

Your HIM department at Pine Valley Community Hospital accepts students as part of their professional practice experience (PPE). Your HIM director wants the confidentiality statement that students sign before they begin their PPE reviewed and updated, if necessary. She has asked you to review the current policy below and suggest modifications for her approval. You decide to research AHIMA resources related to PPE and information security to ensure relevant areas are addressed in the confidentiality statement. Review the policy and make the appropriate modification recommendations.

PINE VALLEY COMMUNITY HOSPITAL PPE CONFIDENTIALITY AGREEMENT

Pine Valley Community Hospital (PVCH) values protection of confidential information concerning patients, their families, medical staff, co-workers, and hospital operations as well. PVCH and the student signing this agreement agree to protect the privacy and security of Protected Health Information (PHI) ensuring compliance with the Health Insurance Portability and Accountability Act of 1996 (HIPAA) and any other applicable laws. The student is obligated to maintain the confidentiality and privacy of PHI throughout their professional practice experience (PPE).

Regardless of how patient and hospital information is stored (paper or computer systems), it is considered confidential. Access to computer systems will be regulated through the use of security codes and confidential passwords. Those individuals granted access are responsible, ethically and legally, to follow the confidentiality requirements and agree to the following:

1. Protect all patient and hospital information

2. Release only authorized information

3. Not to disclose security codes or use another individual's security code

4. Not to write down or otherwise make password or security code accessible

5. Recognize my security code is my electronic signature

I have read and agree to adhere to the conditions of this confidentiality agreement.

_____   _____

Student Signature   Date

_____   _____

Name (Please Print)   Agency/School

Resources

AHIMA. n.d. Professional Practice Experience Guide. Version V. Accessed 21 June 2019. https://www
.ahima.org/ppe.

Miaoulis, W. M. 2014. Practice Brief: Information security—an overview (2014 update). http://bok
.ahima.org/doc?oid=300244#.XE3heFVKi70.

2.22 Encryption

Competency II.2

Competency II.3

The physician practice group you work for is looking for the most secure type of encryption to employ. None of the physicians are familiar with the similarities and differences between symmetric and asymmetric encryption. Compare and contrast the different encryption methodologies for the physicians. Based on the information, provide a recommendation for which methodology you would choose and why.

Resources

Lee-Eichenwald, S. 2020. New Health Information Technologies. Chapter 12 in *Health Information Management: Concepts, Principles, and Practice*, 6th ed. P. Oachs and A. Watters, eds. Chicago: AHIMA.

Sayles, N. B. and L. Kavanaugh-Burke. 2018. *Introduction to Information Systems for Health Information Technology*, 3rd ed. Chicago: AHIMA.

2.23 Authentication

Competency II.2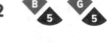

Competency II.3

You have outsourced your emergency department coding to an independent contractor who will be working remotely. Your IT department is requiring a two-factor authentication method for that contractor as an added layer of security. Evaluate the options that you have (use of passwords, tokens, biometrics, or telephone call back) and make a method recommendation supporting your choice.

Resources

Brinda, D. and A. Watters. 2020. Data Privacy, Confidentiality, and Security. Chapter 11 in *Health Information Management: Concepts, Principles, and Practice*, 6th ed. P. Oachs and A. Watters, eds. Chicago: AHIMA.

Lee-Eichenwald, S. 2020. Health Information Technologies. Chapter 12 in *Health Information Management: Concepts, Principles, and Practice*, 6th ed. P. Oachs and A. Watters, eds. Chicago: AHIMA.

Sayles, N. B. and L. Kavanaugh-Burke. 2018. *Introduction to Information Systems for Health Information Technology*, 3rd ed. Chicago: AHIMA.

2.24 Release of information policy

Competency II.1

Competency II.3

In recent weeks, release of information (ROI) clerks have raised questions regarding the release of minors' information. As lead ROI clerk, you have been asked by the HIM department director to compose a procedure that addresses a minor's release of information to adoptive parents, biological parents of adopted minors, noncustodial parents, foster parents, and to an emancipated minor. Create that procedure for each type of release and note whether or not releasing information is appropriate.

Resource

Brodnik, M. S. 2017. Access, Use, and Disclosure and Release of Health Information. Chapter 15 in *Fundamentals of Law for Health Informatics and Information Management*, 3rd ed. M. S. Brodnik, L. A. Rinehart-Thompson, and R. B. Reynolds, eds. Chicago: AHIMA.

2.25 Retention and destruction

Competency II.3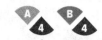

Following are several scenarios related to health record retention and destruction. Draw a conclusion for each scenario, based on health information guidelines, regulations, or best practices.

1. Your organization keeps paper records for ten years, and you are purging records for destruction. What concern do you have with staff pulling records based strictly on that ten-year indicator?

2. Your HIM department is moving to a new office. In the moving process, in the back of a storage closet, a box of old registries is found. These contain records of births at the organization 50 years ago. What should be done with those records?

3. There has been debate in your HIM department about how long fetal monitoring strips must be retained. They are considered part of the mother's health record. What is your recommendation?

4. You have just taken a new job at a tertiary care facility after working in a small community hospital. At your previous place of employment, records were retained for 15 years and then destroyed. At this new facility, records are maintained permanently. What inference can you draw from this difference in procedure?

5. You have just become HIM director at a small critical access hospital. The hospital purges records for destruction quarterly, and the staff has all the records boxed and ready to go. The destruction company workers arrive to collect the records and load them into the truck. They are preparing to leave, but you stop them. Why?

Resource

Rinehart-Thompson, L. A. 2017. Legal Health Record: Maintenance, Content, Documentation, and Disposition. Chapter 9 in *Fundamentals of Law for Health Informatics and Information Management,* 3rd ed. M. S. Brodnik, L. A. Rinehart-Thompson, and R. B. Reynolds, eds. Chicago: AHIMA.

2.26 Network security procedures

Competency II.2

The coding manager at Oak Ridge Memorial Hospital wants to send his coding staff home to work remotely. During discussions with his HIM director, several concerns were raised, including how best to protect patient data while using internet connectivity, whether there are ways to limit access to non-work-related websites, and what to do if an unauthorized person in the home tries to access the hospital's system. The coding manager reaches out to you, an IT professional, to see if there are options that can address these concerns. Recommend technology that can be employed to mitigate these areas of concern and share how they achieve their goals.

Reference

Sayles, N. B. and L. Kavanaugh-Burke. 2018. *Introduction to Information Systems for Health Information Technology*, 3rd ed. Chicago: AHIMA.

Chapter 3

Domain III: Informatics, Analytics, and Data Use

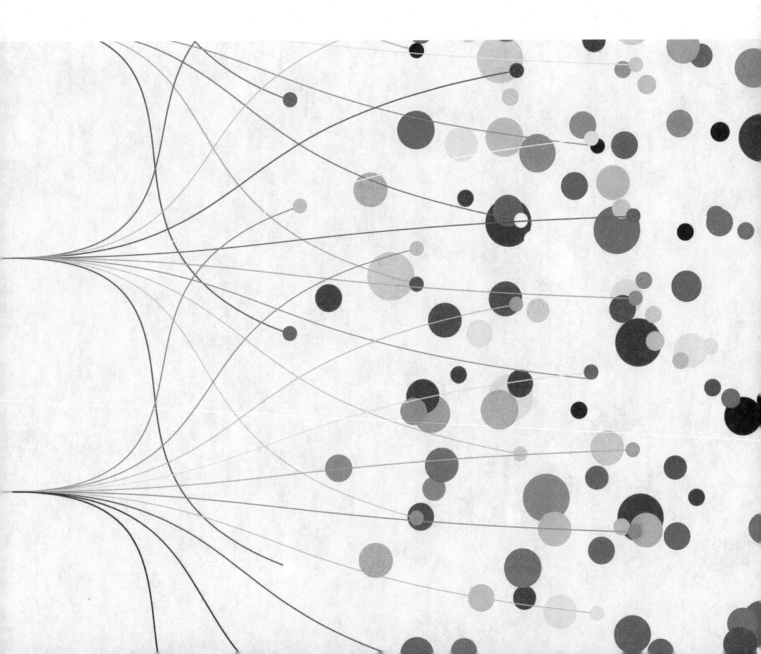

3.0 Inpatient census days

Competency III.3

The HIM director for Pine Valley Community Hospital, which is a critical access hospital, verifies the inpatient service day calculations done by the nursing staff daily.

On Thursday, the census began with 17 inpatients. Of those patients, two were discharged, and one died. Then, four patients were admitted, with one admitted at 9:00 a.m. and then transferred to another facility at 4:00 p.m.

The nursing staff reported 17 inpatient service days. The HIM director is reporting 18.

Compare nursing staff and HIM director reporting. Based on this comparison, who is correct and why?

Resource

Horton, L. A. 2017. *Calculating and Reporting Healthcare Statistics,* 5th ed. revised reprint. Chicago: AHIMA.

3.1 Average daily census

Competency III.3

Competency III.6

As HIM director of West General Hospital, you have been asked to supply the following statistics based on the inpatient service days for the first quarter of this year (non-leap year). Your facility has 150 adult beds, 15 pediatric beds, and 20 bassinets.

West General Community Hospital Inpatient Service Days 1st Quarter 20XX

West General Community Hospital Inpatient Service Days 1st Quarter 20XX	
Type of Service	**Service Days**
Adult	10,430
Pediatric	1,077
Newborn	1,505

1. What was the average daily census for newborns in the first quarter? (Round to nearest whole number)

2. What was the average daily census for adults and children in the first quarter? (Round to the nearest whole number)

Reference

Horton, L. A. 2017. *Calculating and Reporting Healthcare Statistics,* 5th ed. revised reprint. Chicago: AHIMA.

3.2 Bed occupancy rate and change

Competency III.3

Competency III.6

The chief of pediatrics at West General Hospital is interested in the bed occupancy rate for the pediatric unit for the first quarter of the non-leap year. Use the data from exercise 3.1 to complete the following calculations and round each answer to one decimal point.

1. Obtain the pediatric unit's bed occupancy rate.

2. How does the bed occupancy rate for the pediatric unit alone compare with the overall (adults and pediatric patients) bed occupancy rate for the facility?

3. If the bed count in January was 10 beds and the count changed on February 1st to 15 beds for the remainder of the quarter, calculate the change in the pediatric bed occupancy rate.

Resource

Horton, L. A. 2017. *Calculating and Reporting Healthcare Statistics,* 5th ed. revised reprint. Chicago: AHIMA.

3.3 Length of stay/average length of stay

Competency III.3

The HIM director for Pine Valley Community Hospital, a critical access hospital, was reviewing the length of stay for recently discharged patients. The following table lists the discharges for the last two weeks of May.

- Calculate the length of stay for each discharge.
- Calculate the total length of all the stays.
- Calculate the average length of stay for all discharges.

Pine Valley Community Hospital		
Length of Stay		
Date Admitted	Date Discharged	Length of Stay
5/14	5/14 (died)	
5/14	5/17	
5/14	5/21	
5/15	5/21	
5/15	5/18	
5/16	5/21 (died)	
5/16	5/21	
5/17	5/21	
5/17	5/21	
5/18	5/28	
5/18	5/22	
5/18	5/22	
5/19	5/19	
5/19	5/21	
5/20	5/28	
5/21	5/22	
5/22	5/28	
5/23	5/28	
5/23	5/28	
5/24	6/4	
Total		

Resource

Horton, L. A. 2017. *Calculating and Reporting Healthcare Statistics,* 5th ed. revised reprint. Chicago: AHIMA.

3.4 Healthcare statistics

Competency III.3

Based on the data that follows, solve for the answer to the following questions. Round answers to two decimal places unless otherwise directed.

1. What is the adults and children inpatient nosocomial infection rate for the hospital?

2. What was the anesthetic death rate?

3. If the facility's maternal death rate was reported as 0.15%, is that accurate? Support your answer.

4. Would a reported fetal death rate of 0.1% be correct? Support your answer.

5. Is a post-operative infection rate of 0.4% correct? Support your answer.

Lakewood Community Hospital					
Admissions			**Discharges (not including deaths)**		
	Total adults and children	5,359		Total adults and children	5,315
	Total live births	697		Total newborns	699
Infections:			**Included in discharges:**		
	Post-operative	11		OB delivered	1,204
	Inpatient nosocomial			OB aborted	68
	Adults and children	8		OB undelivered, prepartum	12
	Newborn	1		OB undelivered, postpartum	19
			Deaths		
				Total adult and children	16
				Total newborns	3
Total surgical operations		2,721	**Included in death:**		
Total patient operated on		2,715		Within 10 days post-op	1
Total anesthetics administered		2,715		<48 hours after admission	3
				≥48 hours after admission	12
				Anesthetic deaths	1
				Post-operative	4
				Obstetric deaths:	
				Delivered	2
				Undelivered, prepartum	1
				Aborted	2
				Fetal deaths:	
				Early	3
				Intermediate	3
				Late	1

Resource

Horton, L. A. 2017. *Calculating and Reporting Healthcare Statistics,* 5th ed. revised reprint. Chicago: AHIMA.

3.5 IT audit

Competency III.1

As Pine Valley Community Hospital's IT director, management has come to you with concerns of noticeable productivity decline and managers have reported an increase in web surfing. You run random employee audits for the past three months and discover a significant increase in the number of non–work-related websites that are being accessed, such as Facebook, Ticketmaster, and QVC. Propose to your CEO a simple IT solution that could prevent this access. Include a variety of different ways that the solution could be effective.

Resource

Sayles, N. B. and L. Kavanaugh-Burke. 2018. *Introduction to Information Systems for Health Information Technology*, 3rd ed. Chicago: AHIMA.

3.6 Electronic signature

Competency III.1

Competency III.2

A physician has asked your opinion regarding electronically signing his reports. He knows that his EHR will support digital, digitized, and electronic signatures, but he needs clarification about the differences. Give your opinion about which type of signature to use and justify your selection.

Resource

Sayles, N. B. and L. Kavanaugh-Burke. 2018. *Introduction to Information Systems for Health Information Technology*, 3rd ed. Chicago: AHIMA.

3.7 Coding intranet

Competency III.1

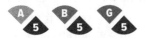

1. As coding supervisor, you have requested and received permission to establish an intranet specifically for coding staff. Recommend elements to include on the site.

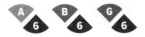

2. Create a screen design for the items you have selected.

Resource

Sayles, N. B. and L. Kavanaugh-Burke. 2018. *Introduction to Information Systems for Health Information Technology*, 3rd ed. Chicago: AHIMA.

3.8 Research methodology

Competency III.5

Six months ago, your multi-system organization implemented computer-assisted coding at one of its campuses. Before you roll it out at another facility, you need to find out how the process is going. Reports indicate that most coders are not making use of the computer-generated codes and are still using the old process for code assignment. It is clear that you will have to do some research to find out what the issues are. Select the research methodology approach best suited for this and defend your choice.

Resources

Houser, S. 2020. Research Methods. Chapter 18 in *Health Information Management: Concepts, Principles, and Practice*, 6th ed. P. Oachs and A. Watters, eds. Chicago: AHIMA.

Watzlaf, V. and E. J. Forrestal. 2017. Research Designs and Methods. Chapter 1 in *Health Informatics Research Methods*, 2nd ed. Chicago: AHIMA.

3.9 Literature review (Medline)

Competency III.5

The chief of obstetrics and gynecology has requested your help with some research. She is hoping to initiate single-site robotic hysterectomies at your hospital. However, administration is requesting details about the procedure, including its safety and how it compares to standard laparoscopic hysterectomy.

1. Make use of Medline to find at least five relevant articles that will assist the OB-GYN chief in making her case with administration. Present your answers in the bibliographic format your instructor specifies.

2. Annotate each article, explaining why you chose to include the article in the literature review.

Resources

Houser, S. 2020. Research Methods. Chapter 18 in *Health Information Management: Concepts, Principles, and Practice*, 6th ed. P. Oachs and A. Watters, eds. Chicago: AHIMA.

Watzlaf, V. and E. J. Forrestal. 2017. Defining the Research Question and Performing a Literature Review. Chapter 10 in *Health Informatics Research Methods*, 2nd ed. Chicago: AHIMA.

3.10 Informed consent—institutional review board

A

B

Competency III.5

Because of your HIM background, your pregnant cousin has emailed you a copy of the informed consent that she received regarding participation in a research study on gestational diabetes. She is unfamiliar with this type of document and wants to be sure it addresses all aspects that it should. Assess the document based on the criteria for research informed consents and provide her with your opinion. Be sure to defend your judgment.

Research on the topic of Gestational Diabetes Management

You are invited to participate in a research study examining the effects of Metformin in the treatment of gestational diabetes. The decision to engage in participation or not is strictly yours. This study plans to address the correlation between the use of Metformin and the effect it may have on the fetus.

Participants will engage in a double-blind research study. You will take a medication to treat your gestational diabetes and will have regular follow-up appointments with our team of physicians, as will your infant after birth. This study will begin at the onset of the gestational diabetes diagnosis and follow you through the first year of the infant's life.

Your participation in the study may be terminated at the discretion of the investigators without your consent. Risks that may be associated with the study include:

- Adverse effects of the medications

The benefit from this research may include control of your gestational diabetes, but there is no guarantee. Women who become pregnant in the future and their children may benefit from the information obtained from this study. Results of significance will be shared with test subjects as the study progresses.

Medications will be provided free of charge while participating in this study. Physician visits for the infant will be covered monthly after delivery. Mileage to these visits will be paid.

Your participation in this research study is voluntary. There is no requirement to participate or to continue participation once you have started. You will incur no penalty nor lose any benefits that you are entitled to if you decide to terminate your participation. Your relationship with our health network will not suffer as a result of termination.

You may call J. Jackson at 999-999-9999 or email J. Jackson at J.Jackson@health.hlt with any questions that you have. This includes questions regarding the study, or questions regarding physical or psychological issues that are developing which you believe to be unusual or unexpected.

CONSENT OF SUBJECT
(or Legally Authorized Representative)

_____   _____
Signature of Subject or Representative   Date

Resources

Harman, L. B. 2017. Research and Ethics. Chapter 14 in *Health Informatics Research Methods*, 2nd ed. V. Watzlaf and E. J. Forrestal, eds. Chicago: AHIMA.

Sandefer, R. 2020. Biomedical and Research Support. Chapter 19 in *Health Information Management: Concepts, Principles, and Practice*, 6th ed. P. Oachs and A. Watters, eds. Chicago: AHIMA.

3.11 AHIMA Foundation research

A

B

Competency III.5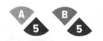

Read the article "The Growth in the Clinical Documentation Specialist Profession" from the AHIMA Foundation's online research journal, *Educational Perspectives in Health Informatics and Information Management* (Barnhouse and Rudman 2013).

1. Determine the research methodology used for the data collection on this topic. Defend this choice of methodology.

2. Interpret the response rate for this data collection and give your opinion regarding its significance.

3. What factors impact response rate, and how might those factors influence the results?

Reference

Barnhouse, T. and W. Rudman. 2013. The growth in the clinical documentation specialist profession. *Educational Perspectives in Health Informatics and Information Management*. http://eduperspectives .ahima.org/the-growth-in-the-clinical-documentation-specialist-profession/.

Resources

Forrestal, E. J. 2017. Selecting the Research Design and Method and Collecting Data. Chapter 11 in *Health Informatics Research Methods*, 2nd ed. V. Watzlaf and E. J. Forrestal, eds. Chicago: AHIMA.

Houser, S. 2020. Research Methods. Chapter 18 in *Health Information Management: Concepts, Principles, and Practice*, 6th ed. P. Oachs and A. Watters, eds. Chicago: AHIMA.

3.12 Institutional review board—vulnerable populations

Competency III.5

As the new director of HIM for Oak Ridge Regional Hospital, one of your duties is to serve as a resource for the Institutional Review Board (IRB). You reviewed their policies and procedures to familiarize yourself with the IRB's functions and are concerned when you do not find any mention of "vulnerable subjects." As you prepare for a meeting with the IRB, what recommendations will you make about addressing vulnerable subjects, and how will you defend your position?

Resources

Sandefer, R. 2020. Biomedical and Research Support. Chapter 19 in *Health Information Management: Concepts, Principles, and Practice*, 6th ed. P. Oachs and A. Watters, eds. Chicago: AHIMA.

Watzlaf, V. and E. J. Forrestal. 2017. Research and Ethics. Chapter 14 in *Health Informatics Research Methods*, 2nd ed. Chicago: AHIMA.

A

B

3.13 Health information exchange models

Competency III.7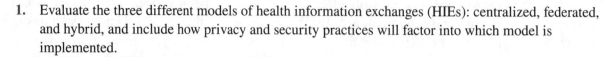

1. Evaluate the three different models of health information exchanges (HIEs): centralized, federated, and hybrid, and include how privacy and security practices will factor into which model is implemented.

2. Evaluate the opt-in and opt-out selections for patients as they relate to HIEs and justify your opinion on which selection has the better chance for success and why.

Resources

AHIMA Thought Leadership Series. 2012. Ensuring Data Integrity in Health Information Exchange. http://library.ahima.org/xpedio/groups/public/documents/ahima/bok1_049675.pdf.
AHIMA. 2013. Understanding the HIE landscape. *Journal of AHIMA* 84(1):56–63.

3.14 Health information exchange policies and procedures

Competency III.7DM

Competency III.7

A health information exchange (HIE) is being established in your area and there are openings for individuals with an HIM background. You learn that one of the primary tasks will be writing policies and procedures. This interests you, but you are unsure what policy topics might need to be addressed. Discover at least five policy topics that an HIM professional could contribute to in an HIE setting by conducting on-line research using AHIMA resources. Supply at least two sources of information.

References

AHIMA. 2015. Policy and Procedure Considerations for Health Information Exchange Organizations. *Journal of AHIMA* 86(8):36–39.

AHIMA. 2011. HIE management and operational considerations. *Journal of AHIMA* 82(5):56–61.

A

3.15 Health information exchange challenges

Competency III.7DM

Competency III.7

As an HIM professional, you have been asked to take part in an open community forum regarding health information exchanges (HIEs). You are anticipating that there will be questions about the challenges that HIE adoption faces, which include the ability to support new payment models.

1. Prepare for these questions first by identifying at least three other HIE challenges.

2. Appraise how to explain that HIEs will support new payment models such as a value-based purchasing.

Resource

Berry, K. 2013. HIE quality check. *Journal of AHIMA* 84(2):28–32.

3.16 Health information exchange and data integrity

Competency III.6

Competency III.7DM

Competency III.7

Suppose you are an HIM professional employed at a health information exchange with 25 component organizations and you see the following report. Discuss these results relative to data integrity. Propose at least five steps to remediate the issue.

MRN	SSN	Last Name	First Name	Middle	DOB	Payment
47233	546-23-XXXX	Baker Sr.	Louis	Howard	5/18/1954	Medicaid
158237	315-24-XXXX	Watson	Michelle	Lee	7/22/1942	Medicare
520613	588-32-XXXX	Jones	Lynn	Tara	10/12/1963	Commercial
723341	213-22-XXXX	Harris	Ann	Marie	9/10/1952	Self
894231	588-32-XXXX	Jones	Tara	Lynn	10/21/1963	Commercial
189011	533-44-XXXX	Marshall	Tucker	B.	11/4/1961	Commercial
218220	151-24-XXXX	Leonard	Timothy	Allen	6/17/1943	Medicare
797536	213-22-XXXX	Harris-Smythe	Ann	Marie	9/10/1952	Commercial
36524	315-24-XXXX	Watson	Michelle	Lee	7/22/1924	Medicare
466100	546-23-XXXX	Baker	Louis	Howard	5/18/1945	Medicare
744183	626-26-XXXX	Baker	Louis	Howard	4/18/1965	Commercial
118231	641-58-XXXX	Thomas	Paul	Carlson	1/16/1971	Self
237352	641-58-XXXX	Carlson	Thomas	Paul	1/16/1971	Self
898233	213-22-XXXX	HarrisSmythe	Ann	Marie	9/1/1952	Commercial
789321	151-24-XXXX	Allen	Timothy	Leonard	6/17/1934	Medicare
664455	213-22-XXXX	SmytheHarris	Ann	Marie	9/1/1925	Commercial
98723	315-42-XXXX	Watson	Michelle	Lee	7/22/1924	Medicare
587532	546-23-XXXX	Baker	Howard	Louis	5/18/1954	Medicaid

Resource

Landsbach, G. and B. Just. 2013. Five risky HIE practices that threaten data integrity. *Journal of AHIMA* 84(11):40–42.

3.17 System testing

Competency III.6

Your information technology department has several system applications due to go live at the same time. They have asked you, the coding supervisor, to move up the installation of your encoder to help them free up some time. No testing has been done yet with the new encoder. Defend your position to wait until the testing is complete to proceed with the installation.

Resource

Sayles, N. B. and L. Kavanaugh-Burke. 2018. *Introduction to Information Systems for Health Information Technology*, 3rd ed. Chicago: AHIMA.

3.18 Data normalization

Competency III.6

At the newly constructed Oak Ridge Regional Hospital, you are working on a team to establish data normalization standards. The process begins by making a normalization decision on patient demographic data. The following information was provided as an example:

Margaret C. Whitfield (Johnson)

123 North West Street, Pine Valley, OH 44444

62 years old, 10/13/52

Blue Cross/Blue Shield 123 East Market St., Lansing, MI 55555

1. How would you recommend the data be normalized?

2. A colleague on the committee thinks the team is wasting time on this process. He does not understand why it matters if the data is normalized or not. Share the organization's motivation for ensuring that data is normalized.

Resource

Sayles, N. B. and L. Kavanaugh-Burke. 2018. *Introduction to Information Systems for Health Information Technology*, 3rd ed. Chicago: AHIMA.

3.19 Desktop versus laptop computers

Competency III.1

As office manager for the new Oakmont Physician Group, you are trying to get all physicians to utilize laptops for office use to facilitate care and reduce costs. Two of the group's physicians prefer desktop computers because they are concerned about laptop security. Defend your recommendation by supplying at least five security features that can be undertaken with laptops to heighten security.

Resource

Herzig, T. 2012. Practice Brief: Mobile device security (2012 update). *Journal of AHIMA* 83(4):50–55.

3.20 Thin client

Competency III.1

At a morning meeting, Joe, the information technology manager of the newly formed Oakmont Physician Group, announced that he wants to initiate a thin client or server network for the practice. One of the physicians approaches you after the meeting and asks you to educate her on what that means. Provide an explanation to help her understand that concept. Also, provide a comparison of the pros and cons of using a thin client server network for the practice.

Resource

Amatayakul, M. K. 2017. *Health IT and EHRs: Principles and Practice*, 6th ed. Chicago: AHIMA.

3.21 Denial dashboard

Competency III.3

Competency III.4

The denial management coordinator at Pine Valley Community Hospital provides the administration with the following dashboard information monthly. As the revenue cycle manager for the facility, you also receive a copy of this dashboard. Formulate four questions that you would have as a result of studying this dashboard and provide the rationale for your questions.

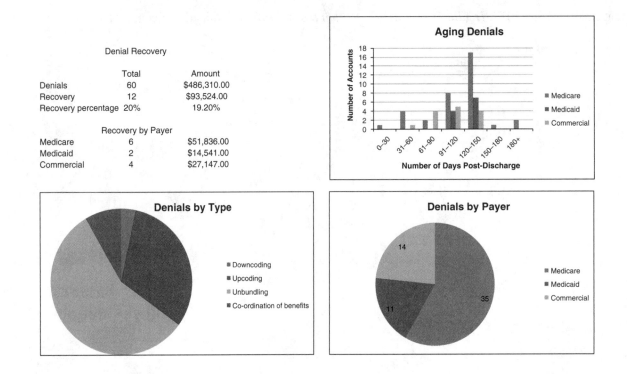

Denial Recovery

	Total	Amount
Denials	60	$486,310.00
Recovery	12	$93,524.00
Recovery percentage	20%	19.20%

Recovery by Payer

Medicare	6	$51,836.00
Medicaid	2	$14,541.00
Commercial	4	$27,147.00

Resource

Handlon, L. 2020. Revenue Cycle Management. Chapter 8 in *Health Information Management: Concepts, Principles, and Practice,* 6th ed. P. K. Oachs and A. L. Watters, eds. Chicago: AHIMA.

3.22 Database structure

Competency III.1

Competency III.6

Competency III.6DM

As the IT director for a large tertiary care center, you were asked to create a database that will collect patient information for the oncology department. You narrowed your database structure to either a relational or a NoSQL database model. The head of oncology asked that you attend a meeting to elaborate on the ability of these models to meet his team's needs and get their feedback prior to making a final decision. Compose your arguments for each model to share with the oncology team. Make a recommendation for the type of database that would best meet their needs.

Resources

Sayles, N. B. and L. Kavanaugh-Burke. 2018. *Introduction to Information Systems for Health Information Technology*, 3rd ed. Chicago: AHIMA.

Sharp, M. and C. Madlock-Brown. 2020. Data Management. Chapter 6 in *Health Information Management: Concepts, Principles, and Practice*, 6th ed. P. Oachs and A. Watters, eds. Chicago: AHIMA.

3.23 Delivery statistics

Competency III.3

Competency III.4

1. In 2013, the chief of obstetrics became concerned about the C-section rate at Oakwood Memorial Hospital. The national rate for C-section delivery at that time was 32.8 percent. A report at that time provided the following data.

Oakwood Memorial Births	
	2013
Vaginal	332
Cesarean	179
Total	511

   a. Determine if his concern is warranted.

   b. Predict the next course of action by the chief of obstetrics based on this information.

2. In the early months of 2019, the new chief of obstetrics asked for a report from the past six years that shows the vaginal and cesarean births. You supply the following information.

Oakwood Memorial Births						
	2013	**2014**	**2015**	**2016**	**2017**	**2018**
Vaginal	332	350	356	388	391	369
Cesarean	179	206	178	183	168	155
Total	511	556	534	571	559	524

   a. The chief of obstetrics wants to know how her department performs against the current national C-section rate of 32.7 percent. Compile the data to answer her question.

   b. Create a graph to show the C-section rate trend over the past six years.

3. The chief now wants to know if there is any correlation between the number of C-sections and maternal deaths versus those that occur after a vaginal delivery. You take the information from 2018 and compile the following Chi square.

	Maternal Death	**No Maternal Death**	**Total**
Vaginal delivery	1	368	369
C-section delivery	4	151	155
Total	5	519	524

If our null hypothesis is that there is no correlation between delivery method and maternal death, and the result of our Chi square is $p = 0.013$, what interpretation do you give the chief of obstetrics?

Resource

Horton, L. A. 2017. *Calculating and Reporting Healthcare Statistics*, 5th ed., revised reprint. Chicago: AHIMA.

3.24 Critical access hospital length of stay

Competency III.3

Competency III.4

As HIM director for a critical access hospital (CAH), you track the average length of stay (ALOS) for the facility. This is a critical piece of information since CMS requires that a CAH have an annual average length of stay of 96 hours or less per patient.

1. Using the data below, solve for the ALOS for the month of February 2018 and test if it meets the ALOS goal.

2. Calculate the standard deviation for this data.

Length of Stay (in days)	Number of Patients
1	5
2	13
3	23
4	21
5	9
6	3
7	1
8	1
10	1
12	1

3. Using the data below, determine if the facility met the goal for the month of August.

4. Based on the data below, what further action would you propose?

Length of Stay (in days)	Number of Patients
2	6
3	12
4	14
5	10
6	7
7	8
8	16
9	10
10	4
11	2
12	3
15	3
18	4
19	1
20	1

5. Create a control chart to show the ALOS by physician using the data below.

Physician	Number of Patients	Length of Stay (in days)
Dr. Mellendorf	14	75
Dr. Snodgrass	15	82
Dr. Gunion	20	137
Dr. Oliver	38	342
Dr. Joyce	14	88
Total		

6. Suggest at least three reasons that the ALOS requirement was or was not met.

7. Based on the results illustrated on the control chart, predict which actions, if any, should be taken by the organization?

8. Create a control chart to depict the 2018 annual ALOS based on the following information.

Jan	4.12
Feb	3.64
March	3.39
April	4.79
May	5.23
June	3.21
July	3.03
Aug	7.17
Sept	3.77
Oct	4.18
Nov	3.54
Dec	3.89

9. What deductions can you make based on this control chart?

10. The control chart does not indicate if the hospital met the annual goal of an ALOS of four days (96 hours) or less. Using the data given, solve for that answer.

Resource

Horton, L. A. 2017. *Calculating and Reporting Healthcare Statistics,* 5th ed., revised reprint. Chicago: AHIMA.

3.25 Strategic planning

Competency III.2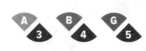

Competency III.6

1. At a recent department head meeting, your organization's CEO indicated that there is discussion about purchasing a lithotripsy machine. What can you assume will be HIM's role in these discussions?

2. You asked your assistant director to run a report for the CEO on the number of patients transferred out for open heart surgery. This is a preliminary investigation to determine if the organization should pursue the expansion of the heart center to include performing open heart surgery. Analyze the following section of the report to identify any errors before you send it on to the CEO.

Patient MRN	Patient Name	Physician	Date of Admission	Date of Discharge	Discharge Disposition
025124	James, T.	Smith	1/3/2015	1/3/2015	X-H
067481	Henderson, P.	Jones	7/22/2015	7/23/2015	X-H
129530	Lewis, J.	Baker	4/15/2015	4/19/2015	X-SNF
088352	Marigold, B.	Conrad	5/12/2015	5/15/2015	X-H
046721	Goodwin, D.	Heller	1/29/2015	1/30/2015	X-H
033799	Summers, T.	Peterson	2/28/2015	3/3/2015	X-NH
080808	Behringer, L.	McMurray	6/23/2015	7/2/2015	X-HO
163540	Lockhart, I.	Campbell	9/12/2015	9/16/2015	X-SNF
118912	Singh, O.	Smith	10/12/2015	10/14/2015	X-H
134577	Packer, W.	Heller	12/1/2015	12/1/2015	X-H
018297	Wade, H.	Jones	4/25/2015	5/1/2015	X-SNF
094722	Lawson, B.	Thompson	10/12/2015	10/13/2015	X-H
075831	Clinger, C.	Smith	11/7/2015	11/8/2015	X-H
039854	DiCesare, D.	Heller	2/3/2015	2/3/2015	X-H
064721	Watson, C.	Peterson	3/18/2015	3/21/2015	X-H
X-H	transfer to hospital				
X-NH	transfer to nursing home				
X-SNF	transfer to skilled nursing home				
X-HO	transfer to hospice				

3. What overall conclusion can you reach about the report?

4. The chief of staff requests a report from HIM on all the patients who have sepsis that died in 2018. Below is a sample of the criteria used to run the report. Evaluate it for accuracy and recommend changes if necessary, justifying your change(s).

Patient Medical Record Number	all
Patient Name	all
Discharge Date	01/01/15–12/13/15
Discharge Disposition	X = expired
MS-DRG	870, 871, 872

Resource

McClernon, S. E. 2020. Strategic Thinking and Management. Chapter 27 in *Health Information Management: Concepts, Principles, and Practice*, 6th ed. P. Oachs and A. Watters, eds. Chicago: AHIMA.

3.26 Release of information tracking log

Competency III.2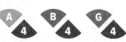

You have been hired as a release of information (ROI) clerk at Oak Wood Memorial Hospital, which has two other ROI clerks. Since starting your job, you are fielding phone calls from a number of angry individuals whose requests were not fulfilled prior to your hire. The current process is to manually log of all the requests for patient information. Without further information, you have no idea if the request was processed or not. You decide to ask for a meeting with the HIM Director to engage in a discussion regarding the benefits of an automated ROI tracking system. Assume that the director is going to need a great deal of persuading in order to consider the purchase of an automated ROI system. What points can you make in your meeting that would support such a system's purchase?

References

Bock, L. J., B. Demster, A. Dinh, E. Gorton, and J. Lantis. 2012. Management Practices for the Release of Information. *Journal of AHIMA* 83(2).

Sayles, N. B. and L. Kavanaugh-Burke. 2018. *Introduction to Information Systems for Health Information Technology*, 3rd ed. Chicago: AHIMA.

3.27 Best of fit versus best of breed

Competency III.2

There has been much discussion in your organization regarding the purchase of an EHR. Two factions are squaring off in the discussions: those that favor best of fit, and those that favor best of breed. The information system (IS) with the backing from IT is a total package with an encoder as part of the system. You have worked with that encoder before and found it to be subpar. Explain why you support the best of breed IS.

Reference

Sayles, N. B. and L. Kavanaugh-Burke. 2018. *Introduction to Information Systems for Health Information Technology*, 3rd ed. Chicago: AHIMA.

3.28 Data analytics—decision support

Competency III.4

As the office manager for a small pediatric group you are reviewing the following dashboard from your information system. The teal lines reflect the actual data, the dark blue line represents the practice's goals.

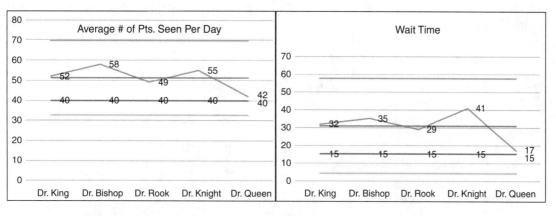

1. What value do these analytics bring to the practice?

2. What one significant action might need to be taken based on this data?

3. What other data would you want to have before taking action?

4. Justify the use of a dashboard as an effective part of a decision-support system.

Resource

Sayles, N. B. and L. Kavanaugh-Burke. 2018. *Introduction to Information Systems for Health Information Technology*, 3rd ed. Chicago: AHIMA.

3.29 Delivery analysis

Competency III.6DM

Competency III.6

The chief of obstetrics is asking for a six-year trend of vaginal versus cesarean section deliveries. You supply the following graph.

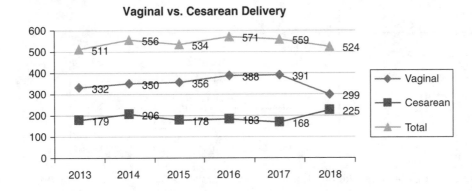

1. Knowing that the national average of C-sections is running at 32.8 percent, what inferences can you make about the hospital's C-section rate based on analysis of this chart?

Using the national average and the hospital C-section rates, you now create this control chart.

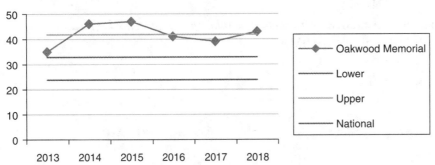

2. What inferences can you make about the organization's cesarean section rate based on analysis of this chart?

Resource

Horton, L. A. 2017. *Calculating and Reporting Healthcare Statistics,* 5th ed., revised reprint Chicago: AHIMA.

3.30 Data warehouse and modeling

Competency III.6

In your role as an IT specialist at your hospital, you have been approached by the chair of the pediatric department to assist in the creation of a database for collection of information on a variety of childhood communicable diseases and vaccination status. You propose using a data warehouse, which would pull information from the hospital's clinical repository. The chairperson is unfamiliar with these terms and asks for clarification.

1. Explain the concept of a data warehouse and differentiate it from a clinical repository.

2. The chairperson states he is familiar with flat file databases and inquires about their use for this project. You state that a relational database may be the better choice. Support your position regarding a relational database being a better choice than a flat file database.

Resources

Amatayakul, M. K. 2017. *Health IT and EHRs: Principles and Practice*, 6th ed. Chicago: AHIMA.

White, S. 2017. Understanding Databases. Chapter 6 in *Introduction to Healthcare Informatics,* 2nd ed. S. Biedermann and D. Dolezel, eds. Chicago: AHIMA.

3.31 Healthcare Effectiveness Data and Information Set report card

Competency III.2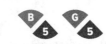

Competency III.6

Your 73-year-old uncle lives in Ohio and is looking for a combined Medicare PPO/HMO to join. Help him create a report card on the healthcare effectiveness data and information set (HEDIS) website to evaluate the health plans. Which health plans should he consider?

Resource

National Committee for Quality Assurance. 2019. Health Plan Report Card. https://reportcards.ncqa.org/#/health-plans/grid?state=Ohio&insurance=Medicare&product=HMO~2FPOS%20Combined.

3.32 Cancer reporting

Competency III.4

As cancer registrar, the cancer committee chairman at your hospital in Napoleon, Ohio, has requested that you create a presentation comparing cancer statistics in the state of Ohio. She wants comparisons among the counties represented by Columbus, Cleveland, Cincinnati, Toledo, and Marietta, along with your own county. You will use the Cancer County Profiles data from Ohio Department of Health website to gather this data.

1. Determine the top three cancer sites by county based on number of cases. Create a table that illustrates this data.

2. Create a bar graph to compare the number of your county's top cancer site cases to the other counties for the same site(s).

3. Use information from the CDC website on cancer statistics to create a graph that compares the percentage of Ohio cancer deaths to total US cancer deaths in 2015 for prostate, lung, colon, and female breast cancers.

Resources

Centers for Disease Control (CDC). 2019 U.S. Cancer Statistics: Data Visualization. https://gis.cdc.gov/cancer/USCS/DataViz.html.

Edgerton, C. 2020. Healthcare Statistics. Chapter 15 in *Health Information Management: Concepts, Principles, and Practice*, 6th ed. P. Oachs and A. Watters, eds. Chicago: AHIMA.

Geology.com. 2019. Ohio County Map with County Seat Cities. http://geology.com/county-map/ohio.shtml.

Ohio Department of Health. 2019. 2015 County Cancer Profiles. http://publicapps.odh.ohio.gov/EDW/DataBrowser/Browse/StateLayoutLockdownCancers

Ohio Department of Health. 2018. Ohio Annual Cancer Report 2018. https://odh.ohio.gov/wps/portal/gov/odh/know-our-programs/ohio-cancer-incidence-surveillance-system/resources/ohio-annual-cancer-report-2018.

3.33 Blockchain

A

B

G

Competency III.1

Competency III.2

1. Sheila Nugent, the IT director at Elmhurst Hospital, is very progressive. She is always assimilating information on the newest technologies to help keep the hospital's records secure while promoting interoperability. Sheila recently began hearing the buzz about blockchain and decided to investigate the topic. Determine what blockchain is and how it can affect interoperability.

2. Sheila thinks blockchain could be a sound investment for the facility with potential for cost-savings; however, she knows the CEO and CFO will require convincing. Sheila understands that many facility investment decisions are based on the bottom line, meaning not only what will the new investment will cost, but also what it will save.

    Sheila decides to speak with Elaine Montgomery, the HIM director. Elaine is also very progressive, and she and Sheila have worked together successfully on several past projects. Sheila is hoping that with Elaine's support, she can convince administrators that blockchain is an IT avenue worth pursuing. Sheila asks Elaine to assess how blockchain technology could affect the revenue cycle, aware it might sway the administrators' position. Provide a detailed assessment that can be used to support the use of this technology.

3. Elaine's biggest concern regarding blockchain technology relates to privacy and security of patient records. How can Sheila persuade Elaine that blockchain technology would not present a privacy or security concern?

Resources

Parks, L. 2019. Is Blockchain Technology in Your Revenue Cycle Future? https://journal.ahima
    .org/2019/02/12/is-blockchain-technology-in-your-revenue-cycle-future/.
Viola, A. 2018. Blockchain's Role in Health IT. *Journal of AHIMA* 89(9): 34–35, 54.

3.34 Contingency plan

Competency III.1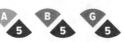

Louis is a recently hired HIM director in a community hospital in Vermont. While reviewing the risk assessment for his department, he is surprised to see that the potential threat of an extended power outage was not addressed. Recent years have brought severe ice storms to the northeastern US that have disrupted power for up to three weeks in some areas. Summer thunderstorms have also been known to wreak havoc on the power supply. This oversight is a big concern to Louis, who begins to develop contingency plans for his department.

One of his major areas of focus is coding, as it will be imperative that accounts continue to be coded so reimbursement continues to flow. While his coding staff work remotely, most of them live within a 25-mile radius of the hospital and are likely to have the same power issues as the facility. Should extreme weather be the cause of an extended power outage, it is likely that most of the staff could report to the hospital once the initial event is over.

Recommend the solutions and alternatives to become part of the contingency plan for this scenario. Be sure to include their benefits and limitations.

Resource

Olenik, K. and R. B. Reynolds. 2017. Security Threats and Controls. Chapter 13 in *Fundamentals of Law for Health Informatics and Information Management,* 3rd ed. M. S. Brodnik, L. A. Rinehart-Thompson, and R. B. Reynolds, eds. Chicago: AHIMA.

A

B

G

3.35 Data analytics

Competency III.1

Competency III.2

Michael is the HIM director for a large primary care physician group in Holmes County, Ohio, which is home to a large Amish population. This group also has a contingent of several pediatricians. Many of the Amish residents in the community come to the group for primary healthcare. Michael is aware of a large measles outbreak going on in the country, which is striking largely unvaccinated populations. He is also aware that within recent years, an Amish community in Ohio suffered from a measles outbreak as well.

After seeing the graph that follows, he is concerned that the outbreak could affect their patients. Analyze how clinical decision support (CDS) software could help identify at-risk patients.

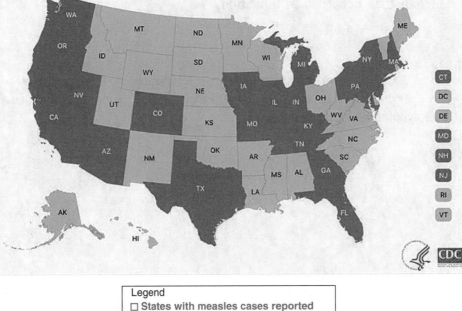

Legend
☐ **States with measles cases reported**
☐ States without measles cases reported

Source: CDC 2019.

Reference

Centers for Disease Control (CDC). 2019. Measles Cases and Outbreaks. https://www.cdc.gov/measles /cases-outbreaks.html.

Chapter 4

Domain IV: Revenue Cycle Management

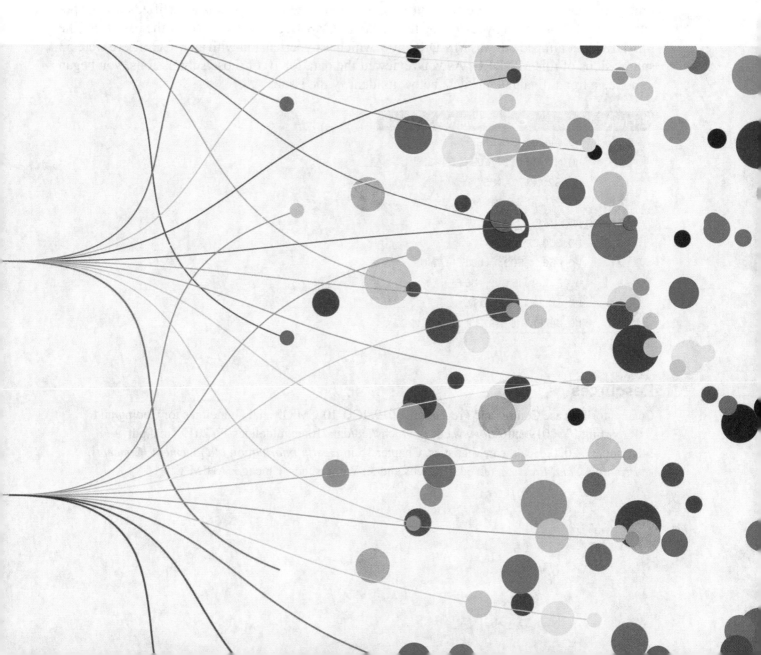

4.0 Case mix issue

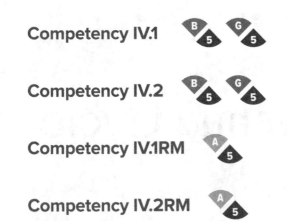

Competency IV.1

Competency IV.2

Competency IV.1RM

Competency IV.2RM

Last year, when you were hired as the HIM director at a small community hospital, the CEO wanted you to focus on increasing the case mix index. The hospital base rate is $7,862. At the time you came on board, there were three coders, only one of whom was a certified coding specialist (CCS). You began by reviewing the number of MS-DRGs submitted over the past year. The MS-DRG that jumped out was MS-DRG 304, which is hypertension with an MCC. There were 53 submissions of this MS-DRG. As you reviewed the data for 10 of those submissions, you began to notice a trend. Evaluate the data below to identify the issue.

Chart	Codes submitted
1	I10, J44.9, N18.6, E11.22
2	I10, N18.6, E10.22, E03.9, G47.33
3	I10, G20, I25.10, N18.5
4	I10, F17.210, I70.213, N18.6, E11.22
5	I10, N18.6, I25.5, I25.10
6	I10, E08.22, N18.6
7	I10, E66.01, E03.9, N18.6, F17.210
8	I10, E87.6, J45.909, N18.6
9	I10, E11.22, E66.9, E78.5, N18.5
10	I10, I25.10, N18.6, R33.9, N18.6, E10.22

Resources

Centers for Disease Control and Prevention. 2019. ICD-10-CM Official Guidelines for Coding and Reporting FY 2019. https://www.cdc.gov/nchs/icd/data/10cmguidelines-FY2019-final.pdf.

Edgerton, C. 2020. Healthcare Statistics. Chapter 15 in *Health Information Management: Concepts, Principles, and Practice*, 6th ed. P. Oachs and A. Watters, eds. Chicago: AHIMA.

4.1 Case mix issue (continued)

Competency IV.2

Competency IV.2RM

Continue using the same information from exercise 4.0.

After reviewing all 53 cases in MS-DRG 304-Hypertension with MCC, you determine that 46 of them have the same error.

Correcting the errors results in reassignment of those cases to a different MS-DRG. Calculate the impact this has on reimbursement by determining the relative weight of the two MS-DRGs and performing the calculations to determine the reimbursement difference.

Resources

Centers for Disease Control and Prevention. 2019. ICD-10-CM Official Guidelines for Coding and Reporting FY 2019. https://www.cdc.gov/nchs/icd/data/10cmguidelines-FY2019-final.pdf.

Edgerton, C. 2020. Healthcare Statistics. Chapter 15 in *Health Information Management: Concepts, Principles, and Practice*, 6th ed. P. Oachs and A. Watters, eds. Chicago: AHIMA.

4.2 Compliance and case mix

Competency IV.2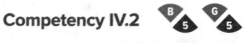

Competency IV.3

Determine the aspects of a compliance plan that need to be addressed following the identification of coding errors such as those that were found in exercise 4.0, and explain why they must be addressed.

Resource

Casto, A. B. 2018. *Principles of Healthcare Reimbursement,* 6th ed. Chicago: AHIMA.

4.3 Inpatient-only procedure denials

Competency IV.1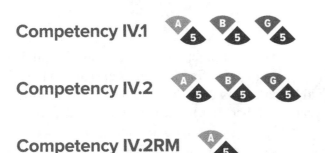

Competency IV.2

Competency IV.2RM

Your organization has a physician who is performing total anterior lumbar arthroplasty with artificial discs on an outpatient basis. Unfortunately, after several have been performed and billed, you get a memo from the business office stating that there are denials for the Medicare patients. The billing manager states that it is something about a status indicator "C." She would like you to review the CPT code assignment(s) and help determine what the problem is and how it can be resolved because the charges for these procedures exceed $65,000 per case.

After reviewing the cases, the CPT code assigned is correct.
*22857–Total disc arthroplasty (artificial disc), anterior approach, including discectomy to prepare interspace (other than for decompression), single interspace, lumbar
*denotes a status indicator of C for that CPT code

1. Explain to the billing manager what status indicator C means.

2. In order to facilitate a prompt resolution to this issue, you and the billing manager decide to create a process improvement team. Decide what hospital departments should be part of the team.

3. Brainstorm at least three possible solutions to the problem.

Resources

Davis, N. A. and B. M. Doyle. 2016. Patient Access. Chapter 4 in *Revenue Cycle Management Best Practices,* 2nd ed. Chicago: AHIMA.

Hazelwood, A. 2020. Reimbursement Methodologies. Chapter 7 in *Health Information Management: Concepts, Principles, and Practice*, 6th ed. P. Oachs and A. Watters, eds. Chicago: AHIMA.

Shaw, P. L. and D. Carter. 2019. Using Teamwork in Performance Improvement. Chapter 4 in *Quality and Performance Improvement in Healthcare,* 7th ed. Chicago: AHIMA.

4.4 Chargemaster process

Competency IV.2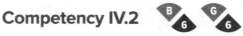

As the new HIM director at Pine Valley Community Hospital, a small critical access hospital, you are surprised to learn that there is no formal process in place for chargemaster maintenance. Requests for additions are supplied by individual departments directly to IT for entry into the chargemaster. No one has deleted any codes for years, and there has never been a systemic review of the chargemaster. You decide to design an improved process for chargemaster maintenance to present to the CEO. Present your newly formulated process in a separate document.

Resources

AHIMA. 2010. Care and maintenance of chargemasters (updated). http://library.ahima.org/xpedio/groups/public/documents/ahima/bok1_047258.hcsp?dDocName=bok1_047258.

Handlon, L. 2020. Revenue Cycle Management. Chapter 8 in *Health Information Management: Concepts, Principles, and Practice*, 6th ed. P. Oachs and A. Watters, eds. Chicago: AHIMA.

4.5 Case management—discharge disposition

Competency IV.2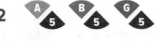

Competency IV.2RM

Your coding staff has been reporting an increase in the number of discharge dispositions that are incorrectly entered in the patients' records in the EHR by case managers. They have to take the time to investigate the correct disposition and make the change, which is causing a decrease in productivity and a corresponding increase in the discharged not final billed total. You have the staff complete a data collection over the next two weeks.

1. Using CMS information, determine the correct discharge status for the seven error types identified based on the information below.

2. Prepare an interpretation of the information and offer recommendations for error reduction to the case manager director.

Coding staff identified the following on review of 198 discharged charts in the two-week period:

- Pine Valley Community Hospital–critical access hospital
- Valley High Children's Hospital–children's hospital
- Valley View Hospital–long-term care hospital
- Big Valley VA Hospital–veteran's affairs hospital
- Valley Vista–inpatient psychiatric hospital

Errors found were:

- 12 transfers to Pine Valley Community Hospital listed as "04."
- 5 transfers to Valley High Children's Hospital listed as "02."
- 7 patients listed as expired "41."
- 3 transfers to Pine Valley Community Hospital swing bed listed as "66."
- 2 patients discharged to jail listed as "10."
- 4 transfers to Valley View Hospital listed as "04."
- 1 transfer to Big Valley VA Hospital inpatient psych unit listed as "65."

Errors by case manager:

- 25 errors by GNF
- 3 errors by MJF
- 6 errors by SWT

Resources

Casto, A. B. 2018. Clinical Coding and Compliance. Chapter 2 in *Principles of Healthcare Reimbursement,* 6th ed. Chicago: AHIMA.

Centers for Medicare and Medicaid Services. 2019. Clarification of patient discharge status codes and hospital transfer policies. https://www.cms.gov/Medicare/Medicare-Contracting/ContractorLearningResources/Downloads/JA0801.pdf.

O'Dell, R. M. 2020. Clinical Quality Management. Chapter 20 in *Health Information Management: Concepts, Principles, and Practice*, 6th ed. P. Oachs and A. Watters, eds. Chicago: AHIMA.

4.6 Utilization review—two-midnight rule

Competency IV.2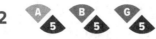

Competency IV.2RM

As HIM director, you have been approached by the utilization review (UR) director to collaborate with her on a presentation for physicians regarding the two-midnight rule as initiated by the Centers for Medicare and Medicaid Services. Review the rule and recommend important information that should be included in the presentation.

Resources

Centers for Medicare and Medicaid Services. 2015. Fact Sheet: Two-midnight Rule. https://www.cms .gov/newsroom/fact-sheets/fact-sheet-two-midnight-rule-0.

Harris, S. L. and J. Kelly. 2015. Building clarity on the two-midnight rule. *Journal of AHIMA* 86(10):68–70.

4.7 Advance beneficiary notice process

Competency IV.2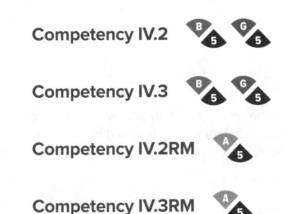

Competency IV.3

Competency IV.2RM

Competency IV.3RM

At a small critical access hospital, individual departments (laboratory, radiology, respiratory therapy) are responsible for issuing an advance beneficiary notice (ABN) for any tests that Medicare may not cover. Other organizations have assigned registration staff the ABN responsibility. Give your opinion on the practice of individual departments issuing ABNs and defend your position.

Resources

Centers for Medicare and Medicaid Services. 2018. Medical Learning Network: Advance Beneficiary Notice of Noncoverage. 4th ed. https://www.cms.gov/Outreach-and-Education/Medicare-Learning-Network-MLN/MLNProducts/downloads/ABN_Booklet_ICN006266.pdf.

Davis, N. A. and B. M. Doyle. 2016. Patient Access. Chapter 4 in *Revenue Cycle Management Best Practices*, 2nd ed. Chicago: AHIMA.

Handlon, L. 2020. Revenue Cycle Management. Chapter 8 in *Health Information Management: Concepts, Principles, and Practice*, 6th ed. P. Oachs and A. Watters, eds. Chicago: AHIMA.

4.8 Resource-based relative value scale

Competency IV.2

Competency IV.2RM

1. Calculate the resource-based relative value scale (RBRVS) payment for a lumbar hemilaminectomy—discectomy performed in each of the cities below using the physician fee schedule search on the CMS website to collect the necessary values. Use the 2018 fee schedule. Create a table to show your work.
    *   Dallas
    *   Chicago
    *   San Francisco
2. Which city has the highest rate? Explain.

Resources

Casto, A. B. 2018. Ambulatory and Other Medicare-Medicaid Reimbursement Systems. Chapter 7 in *Principles of Healthcare Reimbursement,* 6th ed. Chicago: AHIMA.

Centers for Medicare and Medicaid Services. 2019. Physician Fee Schedule Search. https://www.cms.gov/apps/physician-fee-schedule/.

4.9 Accounts receivable days

Competency IV.2 B5 G5

As revenue cycle manager, you oversee the all revenue processes. You just received the report that follows.

	Pine Valley Community Hospital A/R Report March 31, 2019							
	Days Outstanding							
Account Number	Patient Name	Current	30-60	61-90	91-120	121-150	151-180	+180	Total
0013424	Jones		$58.75			$212.15			$270.90
0054261	Williams	$678.50						$6,351.12	$7,029.62
0023789	Matthews	$478.65							$478.65
0052113	Colson			$1,425.97					$1,425.97
0016732	Smith				$653.26				$653.26
0044304	Reynolds		$7,369.82						$7,369.82
0022115	Foster	$682.15		$11,659.72					$12,341.87
0038458	Bell		$5,364.66						$5,364.66
0030071	Brown						$8,416.65		$8,416.65
0021631	Miller		$4,652.31						$4,652.31
0019578	Lockwood	$115.80			$713.48				$829.28
0029824	Johnson		$112.53						$112.53
0043754	Carson	$12,865.40							$12,865.40
0052111	Davis					$311.52			$311.52
0018423	Lawson	$8,789.65							$8,789.65
Totals									
Percentage									

1. Is the patient accounting department meeting the goal of having less than 20 percent of the accounts receivable older than 90 days?

2. Decide what other information may be relevant to capture in this report in order to resolve the outstanding accounts below. Justify inclusion of the proposed information.

3. Should the focus of this report be solely on the oldest accounts? Elaborate on your response.

Resources

Casto, A. B. 2018. Revenue Cycle Management. Chapter 9 *Principles of Healthcare Reimbursement*, 6th ed. Chicago: AHIMA.

Handlon, L. 2020. Revenue Cycle Management. Chapter 8 in *Health Information Management: Concepts, Principles, and Practice*, 6th ed. P. Oachs and A. Watters, eds. Chicago: AHIMA.

4.10 Outpatient Code Editor audit

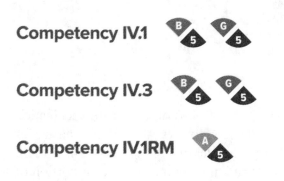

Competency IV.1

Competency IV.3

Competency IV.1RM

Competency IV.3RM

Two months ago, your organization initiated pain management services. In recent weeks, you have watched the accounts receivable for Medicare slowly climbing. You begin to audit the accounts that are outstanding, and realize the reason for the increase is pain management operative procedures, specifically sacroiliac joint injections. These were all billed with CPT code 27096 at approximately $410.00 per case with an average of five cases per day over the past two months. They all have an Outpatient Code Editor (OCE) edit of 28. Determine what your next steps should be to resolve this issue and reduce the accounts receivable.

Resources

Casto, A. B. 2018. Revenue Cycle Management. Chapter 9 in *Principles of Healthcare Reimbursement*, 6th ed. Chicago: AHIMA.

Hazelwood, A. C. 2020. Reimbursement Methodologies. Chapter 7 in *Health Information Management: Concepts, Principles, and Practice*, 6th ed. P. Oachs and A. Watters, eds. Chicago: AHIMA.

4.11 Chargemaster issue

Competency IV.2

Competency IV.2RM

Billing has indicated that they are receiving rejections (OCE edit 28) on Medicare vaccination claims. As the new physician practice manager, you have decided to review the chargemaster for influenza, pneumonia, and hepatitis B vaccination charges to identify the issue(s), since these claims would be hard-coded. The practice sees only adult patients, with a significant portion of them having Medicare as their payer, so it is important to resolve the error(s) quickly. Review the relevant portion of the chargemaster below and revise as necessary. Use the following information in your review:

The hepatitis B vaccines given at this practice are two- or three-dose intramuscular vaccinations. Afluria, Flulaval, Fluvirin, Fluzone, and other not specified flu vaccines are administered to the Medicare population.

Revenue Code	Charge Number	Charge Description	Charge	HCPCS Code	Modifier	CPT code	Status
0252	0682475135	Vaccine-influenza preservative free, IM, 0.25mL	$1.79			90655	Active
0252	0682475136	Vaccine-influenza preservative free, IM, 0.5mL	$2.37			90656	Active
0252	0682475137	Vaccine-influenza IM, 0.25mL	$0.83			90657	Active
0252	0682475138	Vaccine-influenza IM, 0.5mL	$1.32			90658	Active
0252	0693381421	Vaccine-pneumococcal conjugate 7 IM	$5.64			90669	Active
0252	0693381422	Vaccine-pneumococcal conjugate 13 IM	$15.96			90670	Active
0252	0693381423	Vaccine-pneumococcal polysaccharide 23 IM/SQ	$7.89			90732	Active
0771	0753215465	Admin of flu vaccine	$21.75			90471	Active
0771	0753215466	Admin of pneumococcal vaccine	$16.85			90471	Active
0771	0753215467	Admin of hep B vaccine	$19.20			90471	Active

Resources

Casto, A. B. 2018. Revenue Cycle Management. Chapter 9 in *Principles of Healthcare Reimbursement*, 6th ed. Chicago: AHIMA.

Centers for Medicare and Medicaid Services. 2019. Medicare Part B Immunization Billing. https://www.cms.gov/Outreach-and-Education/Medicare-Learning-Network-MLN/MLNProducts/downloads/qr_immun_bill.pdf.

Handlon, L. 2020. Revenue Cycle Management. Chapter 8 in *Health Information Management: Concepts, Principles, and Practice*, 6th ed. P. Oachs and A. Watters, eds. Chicago: AHIMA.

4.12 Chargemaster composition

Competency IV.2

A free-standing radiology facility (Valley Vista Radiology) is being built in your city, and the administrator has contracted with you to help them establish a chargemaster for their services. Examine the portion of their chargemaster illustrated below. Identify the missing elements that should be included for a complete chargemaster and explain their necessity.

Charge Number	Charge Description	Charge	CPT code
0042364527	Chest x-ray, single view	$89.75	71010
0042364528	Chest x-ray, two views	$110.85	71020
0049533561	CT scan, thorax w/o contrast	$450.25	71250
0049533562	CT scan, thorax w/contrast	$525.60	71260
0049533563	CT scan, thorax w/o and w/ contrast	$611.20	71270
0059781213	MRI chest, w/o contrast	$985.00	71550
0059781214	MRI chest, w/contrast	$1,062.65	71551
0059781215	MRI chest, w/o and w/ contrast	$1,145.70	71552

Resources

AHIMA. 2010. Care and maintenance of chargemasters (updated). http://library.ahima.org/xpedio
/groups/public/documents/ahima/bok1_047258.hcsp?dDocName=bok1_047258.

Casto, A. B. 2018. Revenue Cycle Management. Chapter 9 in *Principles of Healthcare Reimbursement,* 6th ed. Chicago: AHIMA.

Handlon, L. 2020. Revenue Cycle Management. Chapter 8 in *Health Information Management: Concepts, Principles, and Practice*, 6th ed. P. Oachs and A. Watters, eds. Chicago: AHIMA.

4.13 Chargemaster requisition form

Competency IV.2

In your role as consultant to Valley Vista Radiology for their chargemaster, you must create a form to be used for future chargemaster requisitions. Determine what elements should be included on the form and then create one to present to the administrator.

Resources

AHIMA. 2010. Care and maintenance of chargemasters (updated). http://library.ahima.org/xpedio /groups/public/documents/ahima/bok1_047258.hcsp?dDocName=bok1_047258.

Casto, A. B. 2018. Revenue Cycle Management. Chapter 9 in *Principles of Healthcare Reimbursement*, 6th ed. Chicago: AHIMA.

Handlon, L. 2020. Revenue Cycle Management. Chapter 8 in *Health Information Management: Concepts, Principles, and Practice*, 6th ed. P. Oachs and A. Watters, eds. Chicago: AHIMA.

Richey, J. 2001. A new approach to chargemaster management. *Journal of AHIMA* 72(1): 51–55.

4.14 Remittance advice

Competency IV.2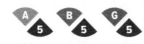

Competency IV.3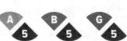

The claim for S. Smith, a 10-year-old that had a tonsillectomy on May 8, 2019, was billed with the following information on May 12, 2019:

S. Smith
123 New Road
Bridgeville, OH 44556
DOB 6/12/1950
CPT code 42825

Claim adjustment reason code (CARC) 6 returned on the remittance advice to indicate the procedure was not paid.

Determine the issue that the CARC identifies and what steps must be taken to correct it.

Resources

Casto, A. B. 2018. Revenue Cycle Management. Chapter 9 in *Principles of Healthcare Reimbursement,* 6th ed. Chicago: AHIMA

X12. 2015. Claim Adjustment Reason Codes. http://www.wpc-edi.com/reference/codelists/healthcare/claim-adjustment-reason-codes/.

4.15 Claim reconciliation

Competency IV.2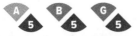

Mrs. Jones had an arthroscopic shoulder procedure on 7/8/19. Her physician performed a subacromial decompression. The coder assigned CPT 29826 to the encounter. The bill dropped on 7/12/19. On 7/22/19, the patient accounting department was processing the latest remittance advice and remark code N122 was attributed to the CPT code for this claim.

1. Determine what the remittance advice remark code (RARC) N122 signifies.

2. Determine the steps needed to correct the claim by utilizing official CPT resources.

Resources

Casto, A. B. 2018. Revenue Cycle Management. Chapter 9 in *Principles of Healthcare Reimbursement*, 6th ed. Chicago: AHIMA.

X12. 2019. Claim Adjustment Reason Codes. http://www.wpc-edi.com/reference/codelists/healthcare/remittance-advice-remark-codes/.

4.16 Electronic data interchange

Competency IV.3

You have just been hired as the revenue cycle manager at a local acute care hospital. One of the first items of business is to review the processes in place for the revenue cycle, and you are surprised to see that no external coding audits have been done for several years. When you ask the coding manager why no external audits have been performed, she explains that the HIM director was told by the director of finance that the cost would not justify the expenditure. You decide to request a meeting with the finance director to present a case defending the need for external audits. Draft a recommendation with your rationale as to the importance of external audits and reasoning for how the expense of external audits can be mitigated.

Resource

Davis, N. A. and B. M. Doyle. 2016. Record Completion and Coding. Chapter 6 in *Revenue Cycle Management Best Practices*, 2nd ed. Chicago: AHIMA.

4.17 Hospital-acquired conditions and present on admission

Competency IV.2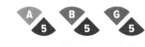

Competency IV.2RM

A 76-year-old morbidly obese white male was admitted to the facility with an acute exacerbation of COPD. He is a previous smoker but has not smoked for the past year because his breathing issues have continued to worsen. He was started on oxygen and treated with an oral corticosteroid with prophylactic antibiotics administered. The progress note for day two states that the pressure ulcer of his right heel (stage 4) was non-excisionally debrided at the bedside.

As an auditor, you review the present on admission (POA) status, code assignment, and DRG assignment shown below for this patient's stay. You conclude there is an error.

POA status	ICD-10-CM codes assigned	DRG assignment 192
Y	J44.1	
N	L89.614	
Y	E66.01	
E	Z87.891	

1. What is the error, and what impact does it have on reimbursement?

2. What action might need to be taken to justify your conclusion of a coding error?

Resources

Casto, A. B. 2018. Value-Based Purchasing. Chapter 9 in *Principles of Healthcare Reimbursement*, 6th ed. Chicago: AHIMA.

Hunt, T. J. and K. Kirk. 2020. Clinical Documentation Improvement and Coding Compliance. Chapter 9 in *Health Information Management: Concepts, Principles, and Practice*, 6th ed. P. Oachs and A. Watters, eds. Chicago: AHIMA.

4.18 Ambulatory payment classification audit

Competency IV.3

Competency IV.3RM

As the physician practice manager, you have run the report with the results depicted in the graph below which shows the distribution of E&M codes billed for established patients over the previous six months.

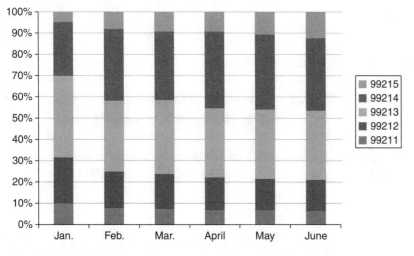

1. What conclusions can you draw from the graph?
2. Recommend four steps that should be taken as a result of your conclusions.

Resources

Casto, A. B. 2018. Clinical Coding and Coding Compliance. Chapter 2 in *Principles of Healthcare Reimbursement*, 6th ed. Chicago: AHIMA.

Hunt, T. J. and K. Kirk. 2020. Clinical Documentation Improvement and Coding Compliance. Chapter 9 in *Health Information Management: Concepts, Principles, and Practice*, 6th ed. P. Oachs and A. Watters, eds. Chicago: AHIMA.

4.19 Claim denial

Competency IV.2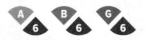

Two patients had a right-posterior subcapsular cataract extraction done with phacoemulsification. An anterior chamber intraocular lens was inserted during the same operative session for both patients. One was done in December of 2014; the other done in February 2015. The 2014 claim was returned with OCE edit 71; while the 2015 claim was returned with OCE edit 92.

- What do the edits mean? Why are they different?
- Create a line item for the chargemaster that will resolve this issue in the future.

Resources

Casto, A. B. 2018. Revenue Cycle Management. Chapter 9 in *Principles of Healthcare Reimbursement,* 6th ed. Chicago: AHIMA.

Centers for Medicare and Medicaid Services. 2019. MLN Matters, MM9005. https://www.cms.gov /Outreach-and-Education/Medicare-Learning-Network-MLN/MLNMattersArticles/downloads /MM9005.pdf.

Handlon, L. 2020. Revenue Cycle Management. Chapter 8 in *Health Information Management: Concepts, Principles, and Practice*, 6th ed. P. Oachs and A. Watters, eds. Chicago: AHIMA.

4.20 Anemia query

Competency IV.3RM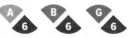

Create a physician query for the following scenario.

A 79-year-old female, Mrs. Carmichael, is admitted on June 15, 2019 with a right hip fracture. Prior to surgery, her attending physician, Dr. Fellows, orders blood work to check her hemoglobin and hematocrit levels because she is borderline anemic. The patient is cleared for surgery with hemoglobin of 12 and hematocrit of 44 percent. Post-surgery, levels are checked again with drop in both to 8 and 32 percent, respectively. The physician orders a blood transfusion of 3 units of packed red cells. In the discharge summary the physician only notes anemia, along with the patient's hip fracture.

Resources

Bossoondyal, S., G. Bryant, T. Combs, et al. 2019. Practice Brief: Guidelines for achieving a compliant query practice. http://bok.ahima.org/doc?oid=302674#.XRd0vetKi70.

Hunt, T. J. and K. Kirk. 2020. Clinical Documentation Improvement and Coding Compliance. Chapter 9 in *Health Information Management: Concepts, Principles, and Practice*, 6th ed. P. Oachs and A. Watters, eds. Chicago: AHIMA.

A

B

G

4.21 Coding error

Competency IV.1RM

Competency IV.1

As the coding manager at a facility in Ohio, you receive accounts from the billing department with potential coding issues prior to billing. It is your job to investigate the account and ensure the proper codes have been assigned. Today, there is a medical necessity edit that has not been cleared concerning Epoetin administration. The codes assigned to this outpatient account were:

First-listed diagnosis   I10
Secondary diagnoses   N18.6
                                    D64.9
                                    E10.9
                                    T82.868A

1. Read the following information from this chart and discuss in detail what the coding error(s) is or are.

2. Modify the coding so that you will be able to clear the medical necessity edit based on the documentation.

Patient Name: Joe Smith   MR#3654777

Acct. # 0000325414   DOS: 10/28/19

Discharge date: 10/29/19

Mr. Smith arrives today with thrombosis of his AV graft. He was unable to receive his dialysis treatment today and will undergo a thrombectomy procedure to restore graft function. He is a 54-year-old with hypertension and diabetes taken to the OR and prepped and draped in the usual sterile fashion. An incision was made permitting access to the graft. A graftotomy was done and Fogarty catheter inserted to pull back the thrombosis. After successful removal of the thrombosis, an injection was performed of the anastomotic area to ensure that the graft was functional. Incision into the graft was then closed, as was the access incision. Patient was taken to the recovery room in stable condition. He will be observed overnight and receive his dialysis tomorrow prior to discharge. He is also to receive an injection of Epoetin for his anemia of CKD.

Resources

Centers for Medicare and Medicaid Services. 2019. Local Coverage Determinations by State Index. https://www.cms.gov/medicare-coverage-database/indexes/lcd-state-index .aspx?bc=AgAAAAAAAAA.

Optum360. 2019. *ICD-10-CM Expert for Hospitals:* The Complete Official Code Set. Salt Lake City: Optum.

4.22 Coding and UHDDS

Competency IV.1RM

Competency IV.1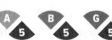

You have agreed to accept an HIM student for their professional practice experience at your facility. Today you are working on coding. You are giving feedback on the codes that the student assigned for the following scenario. Justify and explain the correct coding for this account, by tying your feedback to the Uniform Hospital Discharge Data Set and reimbursement.

Patient: John Smith   MR#121212   Acct. # 000633553

Patient came to ER complaining of chest pain. EKG and labs, including troponin levels, were performed. Nitroglycerin was administered and oxygen therapy initiated. Results of the tests indicated the patient was having an anterior wall myocardial infarction. Patient was taken to the cath lab for immediate single vessel angioplasty. Following the percutaneous coronary intervention, the patient was admitted to the floor. He was monitored continuously. Beta blockers and Coumadin therapy were begun. The patient's hypertension was addressed, and he received medication for low potassium levels as well. His diabetes was managed by medication and diet with no significant issues during the admission. After four days the patient was discharged home to continue his medication regime and begin cardiac rehab.

Codes assigned by student:

Px Dx:	R07.9
	I10
	E87.6
	I21.09
	E11.9
PX Px:	02703ZZ

Resources

Brinda, D. 2020. Data Management. Chapter 6 in *Health Information Management Technology: An Applied Approach*, 6th ed. N. B. Sayles and L. Gordon, eds. Chicago: AHIMA.

Optum360. 2019. ICD-10-CM Expert for Hospitals: The Complete Official Code Set. Salt Lake City: Optum.

A

B

G

4.23 Computer-assisted coding and fraud detection

Competency IV.3

As a coding supervisor, you would like to see computer-assisted coding (CAC) implemented in your organization. You recognize that you will have to convince administrators of the merit of investing in this technology that goes beyond coding. Knowing that compliance has been a major focus of the organization, create a memo to the chief financial officer, Ms. Moneybags, which proposes the use of CAC to assist with fraud detection and prevention.

Resources

Comfort, A., C. D'Amato, C. Isom, T. Rihanek, and D. Thomas-Flowers. 2013. Practice Brief: Automated coding workflow and CAC practice guidance (2013 update). http://bok.ahima.org /doc?oid=300265#.XRd20utKi70.

Eramo, L. A. 2011. Stopping fraud: Detecting and preventing fraud in the e-Health era. *Journal of AHIMA* 82(3):28–30.

4.24 Struggling clinical documentation improvement process

Competency IV.3RM

Competency IV.3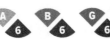

There is one physician at your organization that has seven outstanding queries over the past month; several are more than three weeks old. The queries all regard the clinical validity of an acute blood anemia diagnosis that he has listed on the chart. As revenue cycle manager, you want to get these issues resolved as quickly as possible, so you propose an internal escalation policy. Formulate a proposal to share with your clinical documenation improvement (CDI) and HIM directors for feedback.

Resources

Bossoondyal, S., G. Bryant, T. Combs, et al. 2019. Practice Brief: Guidelines for achieving a compliant query practice. http://bok.ahima.org/doc?oid=302674#.XRd48utKi71.

Brinda, D. 2020. Data Management. Chapter 6 in *Health Information Management Technology: An Applied Approach*, 6th ed. N. B. Sayles and L. Gordon, eds. Chicago: AHIMA.

Denton, D. B., M. Endicott, C. Ericson, T. Love, L. McDonald, and D. Willis. 2016. Clinical Validation: the Next Level of CDI. http://library.ahima.org/PB/ClinicalValidation#.XRd5TutKi70.

4.25 Query retention

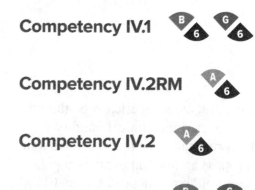

Competency IV.1

Competency IV.2RM

Competency IV.2

Competency IV.3

Your organization is in the process of implementing a clinical documentation improvement (CDI) program. The newly appointed CDI director has made it clear that she is not interested in having input from the HIM department on the program's development. However, in your role as HIM director, someone has made you aware of a CDI policy stating that once a query is answered and the information passed on to the coder, the query form will not be retained.

Consider how to approach the CDI director with your differing opinion on this policy. Be sure to justify the position that you take.

Resources

Bossoondyal, S., G. Bryant, T. Combs, K. DeVault, M. Endicott, C. Ericson, O. Ewoterai, K. Good, T. Grier, W. Haik, T. Hicks, F. Jurack, K. Kozlowski, C. Mogbo, B. Murphy, L. Prescott, S. Schmitz, C. Seluke, S. Wallace, M. Wieczorek, A. Yuen, and I. Zusman. 2019. Practice Brief: Guidelines for achieving a compliant query practice. http://bok.ahima.org/doc?oid=302674#.XRd48utKi71.

Hunt, T. J. and K. Kirk. 2020. Clinical Documentation Improvement and Coding Compliance. Chapter 9 in *Health Information Management: Concepts, Principles, and Practice*, 6th ed. P. Oachs and A. Watters, eds. Chicago: AHIMA.

Sharp, M. 2020. Secondary Data Sources. Chapter 7 in *Health Information Management Technology: An Applied Approach*, 6th ed. N. B. Sayles. and L. Gordon, eds. Chicago: AHIMA.

4.26 Query format

Competency IV.1

Competency IV.2RM

Competency IV.2

Decide if the following is an acceptably formatted physician query and defend your response.

Dr. Hightower

Mrs. Smith was admitted on 8/25, and two days later you mention in a progress note a stage three pressure ulcer of her heel that you debrided at the bedside. Can you clarify was the stage three heel pressure ulcer present on admission?

_____Yes

_____No

C. Coder 9/2

Ext. 2112

Resources

Bossoondyal, S., G. Bryant, T. Combs, K. DeVault, M. Endicott, C. Ericson, O. Ewoterai, K. Good, T. Grier, W. Haik, T. Hicks, F. Jurack, K. Kozlowski, C. Mogbo, B. Murphy, L. Prescott, S. Schmitz, C. Seluke, S. Wallace, M. Wieczorek, A. Yuen, and I. Zusman. 2019. Practice Brief: Guidelines for achieving a compliant query practice. http://library.ahima.org/doc?oid=301357#.XD4velVKi70.

Bowman, S., P. C. Smith, K. DeVault, et al. 2008. Managing an effective query process. _Journal of AHIMA_ 79(10):83–88.

Hunt, T. J. and K. Kirk. 2020. Clinical Documentation Improvement and Coding Compliance. Chapter 9 in _Health Information Management: Concepts, Principles, and Practice_, 6th ed. P. Oachs and A. Watters, eds. Chicago: AHIMA.

Sharp, M. 2020. Secondary Data Sources. Chapter 7 in _Health Information Management Technology: An Applied Approach_, 6th ed. N. B. Sayles and L. Gordon, eds. Chicago: AHIMA.

4.27 Coding audit I

Competency IV.1

Competency IV.3

A coding manager conducted an internal audit of cases in MS-DRG 195 Simple pneumonia without an MCC/CC. There were 619 discharges in this MS-DRG in the previous six months coded by one of five inpatient coders. Twenty-five charts were pulled at random and the coding reviewed with the results noted below. Evaluate the audit process used.

	# of Charts reviewed	MS-DRG change?
Martha	7	1
John	3	0
Samantha	1	1
Karen	12	4
Tom	2	2
Total	25	8

Resources

Gordon, L. 2020. Management. Chapter 17 in *Health Information Management Technology: An Applied Approach*, 6th ed. N. B. Sayles and L. Gordon, eds. Chicago: AHIMA.

Hunt, T. J. and K. Kirk. 2020. Clinical Documentation Improvement and Coding Compliance. Chapter 9 in *Health Information Management: Concepts, Principles, and Practice*, 6th ed. P. Oachs and A. Watters, eds. Chicago: AHIMA.

4.28 Coding audit II

Competency IV.1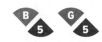

Competency IV.3

Continuing with the case described in 4.27, evaluate the results and recommend next steps.

For convenience, the case scenario and data are repeated below.

A coding manager conducted an internal audit of cases in MS-DRG 195 Simple pneumonia without an MCC/CC. There were 619 discharges in this MS-DRG in the previous six months coded by one of five inpatient coders. Twenty-five charts were pulled at random and the coding reviewed with the results noted below. Evaluate the audit *results* and recommend next steps.

	# of Charts reviewed	MS-DRG change?
Martha	7	1
John	3	0
Samantha	1	1
Karen	12	4
Tom	2	2
Total	25	8

Resources

Gordon, L. 2020. Management. Chapter 17 in *Health Information Management Technology: An Applied Approach*, 6th ed. N. B. Sayles and L. Gordon, eds. Chicago: AHIMA

Hunt, T. J. and K. Kirk. 2020. Clinical Documentation Improvement and Coding Compliance. Chapter 9 in *Health Information Management: Concepts, Principles, and Practice*, 6th ed. P. Oachs and A. Watters, eds. Chicago: AHIMA.

4.29 New staff physician

Competency IV.2

Your organization just hired a new pulmonologist. He has an established practice, and many of his patients are geriatric with advanced COPD, severe asthma, end-stage emphysema, or advanced stage lung cancer. What influence do you expect to see in the organization's case mix index as a result of his hiring and why?

Resources

Casto, A. B. 2018. Medicare-Medicaid Prospective Payment Systems for Inpatients. Chapter 6 in *Principles of Healthcare Reimbursement,* 6th ed. Chicago: AHIMA.

Edgerton, C. G. 2020. Healthcare Statistics. Chapter 16 in *Health Information Management: Concepts, Principles, and Practice*, 6th ed. P. Oachs and A. Watters, eds. Chicago: AHIMA.

Shaw, P. L. and D. Carter. 2019. *Quality and Performance Improvement in Healthcare, A Tool for Programmed Learning,* 7th ed. Chicago: AHIMA.

4.30 Clinical documentation improvement monitoring

Competency IV.2RM

Competency IV.2

In July of 2016, your organization implemented a clinical documentation improvement program. Below is information regarding the quarterly case mix index over the past several years. Discuss the results, theorizing about the fluctuations.

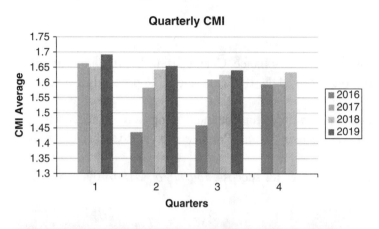

Quarterly Case Mix Index				
	1st Quarter	**2nd Quarter**	**3rd Quarter**	**4th Quarter**
2016		1.4362	1.4587	1.5941
2017	1.6627	1.5829	1.6101	1.5955
2018	1.6518	1.6425	1.6247	1.6340
2019	1.6921	1.6543	1.6401	

Resources

Arrowood, D., L. Bailey-Woods, E. Barnette, T. Combs, M. Endicott, and J. Miller. 2016. *CDI Toolkit*. http://bok.ahima.org/doc?oid=301829.

McNeill, M. H. 2020. Healthcare Statistics. Chapter 14 in *Health Information Management Technology: An Applied Approach*, 6th ed. N. B. Sayles and L. Gordon, eds. Chicago: AHIMA.

4.31 Compliance policy

Competency IV.3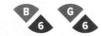

As coding manager, you are seeking approval for an external coding audit to be performed. However, you realize that there is no formal policy in place for this process.

1. Formulate a series of considerations that should be covered in such a policy (provide at least five) to share with your HIM director.

2. Explain why it is important to have a policy in place for an external auditing process.

Resources

Foltz, D. A. and K. Lankisch. 2020. Fraud and Abuse Compliance. Chapter 16 in *Health Information Management Technology: An Applied Approach*, 6th ed. N. B. Sayles and L. Gordon, eds. Chicago: AHIMA.

Hunt, T. J. and K. Kirk. 2020. Clinical Documentation Improvement and Coding Compliance. Chapter 9 in *Health Information Management: Concepts, Principles, and Practice*, 6th ed. P. Oachs and A. Watters, eds. Chicago: AHIMA.

Prophet, S. 1998. Coding compliance: practical strategies for success. *Journal of AHIMA* 69(1):50–61.

4.32 Coding review

Competency IV.1RM

Competency IV.1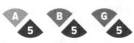

Evaluate the code assignments for the scenario that follows, identifying any errors based on the documentation.

H&P

A 63-year-old woman is admitted with severe, unrelenting headache. CT scan in ER shows an area suspicious for a brain tumor. The woman is admitted to control pain and identify source of primary.

She is a diabetic with hypertension. She smokes a pack of cigarettes a day and has for the past forty years. There is a family history of breast cancer with her aunt and sister.

Patient will undergo an MRI of the brain and CT of chest and abdomen in hopes of identifying primary source of tumor.

Consult

This 63-year-old white female is complaining of numbness and tingling to her feet. She is diabetic, type I, with noncompliance with her insulin treatment. She states that she takes half of the required dosage as it is difficult for her to afford her medications. Examination of extremities is indicative of diabetic neuropathy. Have stressed with the patient the need for her to strictly follow her insulin regimen, and follow up for additional tests as an outpatient. Patient needs to have annual foot and eye exams.

Progress Note I

Patient having CT scans this morning. Will consult with radiology and proceed with recommendations once those results are read.

Progress Note II

Appreciate consult on diabetic management. Will echo consultant's call for compliance with medication.

CT scans showed a right breast lesion, suspicious for malignancy. Patient was informed and is willing to proceed to OR for mastectomy.

CT Report

Patient was given contrast material and CT of the chest performed. A density, consistent with a malignancy was identified in the lower-inner quadrant of the right breast. No abnormalities in the left breast or elsewhere in the chest.

OR Report

Patient was brought to the OR where she was prepped and draped in a sterile manner. She had previously been informed of the risks, benefits, and alternatives to the surgery and elected to proceed.

I made standard mastectomy incisions and dissected down to but not including the pectoral muscle. Bleeders were cauterized and hemostasis secured. The breast was lifted off the musculature. The patient did not want reconstruction at this time, so a primary closure was completed. The specimen was sent to pathology.

Blood loss was minimal and the patient tolerated the procedure well. She is sent to recovery and will be observed until she meets discharge criteria. I will have her follow up in the office in two weeks to discuss treatment of the brain cancer.

Pathology Report

Specimen is 0.3942 kgs. of breast tissue, right breast. Microscopic examination reveals adenocarcinoma.

Discharge Summary

An unfortunate woman who was found to have a breast malignancy (primary) after CT scan identified a metastasis to the brain. She underwent a mastectomy earlier today and is ready for discharge. She will follow up in two weeks to check the healing and discuss further treatment to focus on the brain. She is to follow her medication regimen for diabetes and hypertension. She has been counseled on smoking cessation.

Codes assigned:

C50.911

C71.9

E10.9

I10

F17.210

Z79.4

Z80.3

0HTT0ZZ

Resources

Hazelwood, A. 2020. Reimbursement Methodologies. Chapter 7 in *Health Information Management: Concepts, Principles, and Practice*, 6th ed. P. Oachs and A. Watters, eds. Chicago: AHIMA.

Optum360. 2019. *ICD-10-CM Expert for Hospitals*: The Complete Official Code Set. Salt Lake City: Optum.

Optum360. 2019. *ICD-10-PCS 2019 Expert.* Salt Lake City: Optum.

4.33 National Correct Coding Initiative guidelines

Competency IV.1

Competency IV.3

The billing office manager has emailed you about an issue with patient accounts. They are getting a large number of denials on arthroscopic meniscectomy procedures of the knee for Medicare patients. The denials are related to codes 29880 and 29876 when both codes are billed with modifiers RT, LT, or 50. He is wondering if these denials can be appealed, perhaps by using another modifier. You perform an internal audit of knee arthroscopic meniscectomy procedures and identify the following:

29880 and 29876 are being coded together for the same knee 64 percent of the time with two of your three outpatient coders responsible for these code assignments.

1. Based on NCCI edits, elaborate on the appropriateness of this coding practice and whether or not the denials can be appealed.

2. Develop a process to ensure that NCCI arthroscopy guidelines are followed.

Resources

Casto, A. B. 2018. Revenue Cycle Management. Chapter 9 in *Principles of Healthcare Reimbursement,* 6th ed. Chicago: AHIMA.

Centers for Medicare and Medicaid Services. 2019. *NCCI Policy Manual for Medicare Services.* https://www.cms.gov/Medicare/Coding/NationalCorrectCodInitEd/index.html?redirect= /NationalCorrectCodInitEd/.

Hazelwood, A. 2020. Reimbursement Methodologies. Chapter 7 in *Health Information Management: Concepts, Principles, and Practice*, 6th ed. P. Oachs and A. Watters, eds. Chicago: AHIMA.

4.34 Severity of illness and diagnosis-related groups

Competency IV.2

As a coder transitioning to a new role as a clinical documentation improvement (CDI) specialist, you know about MS-DRGs, but often hear other CDI specialists refer to APR-DRGs. You decide to do a comparison between the two DRG systems in order to understand the similarities and differences.

1. Provide the outcome of your research on MS-DRGs and APR-DRGs.

2. What inferences can you draw from the information you uncovered on these two payment systems in the context of paying for performance?

Resources

Davis, N. A. and B. M. Doyle. 2016. Payer Reimbursement. Chapter 3 in *Revenue Cycle Management Best Practices,* 2nd ed. Chicago: AHIMA.

Hess, P. C. 2015. The Translation of Clinical Documentation in Coded Data. Collecting, Analyzing, and Reporting on Program Data. Chapters 3 and 11 in *Clinical Documentation Improvement: Principles and Practice.* Chicago: AHIMA.

3M. *3M APR DRG Classification System and 3M APR DRG Software Fact Sheet.* http://multimedia.3m.com/mws/media/478415O/3m-apr-drg-fact-sheet.pdf?fn=aprdrg_fs.pdf.

Sturgeon, J. 2013. APR-DRGs in the Medicaid population. *For the Record* 25(5):6.

4.35 MS-DRGs

Competency IV.2

In 2005, there were two DRGs for pneumonia: DRG 89 and DRG 90. In 2007, a revision was made to the DRG system with the result that pneumonia now has three DRGs: 193, 194, and 195. What was the motivation behind the evolution of the DRG payment system and the impact this change had on organizational reimbursement?

Resource

Casto, A. B. 2018. Medicare-Medicaid Prospective Payment Systems for Inpatients. Chapter 6 in *Principles of Healthcare Reimbursement,* 6th ed. Chicago: AHIMA.

4.36 Computer-assisted coding

Competency IV.1RM

Competency IV.1

Competency IV.3RM

Competency IV.3

Your organization is considering using computer-assisted coding (CAC). You create the test case that follows to see how different applications will code the scenario to help you reach a purchase decision.

Mr. Reynolds is a 57-year-old white male admitted with chest pain. He developed this pain while shoveling snow outside his home. He ranks it an 8 out of 10 on the pain scale. He has no arm or jaw pain. He has hyperlipidemia and hypertension, and is on medication for both conditions. Last year, he suffered an acute myocardial infarction and was treated with two coronary stents.

An EKG was performed and cardiac enzymes drawn. All results were normal. The patient exhibited the pain upon movement and palpation at the chondrosternal joint and a final diagnosis of sprain was determined.

Codes assigned by CAC:

R07.9

I21.3

R68.84

S23.421A

I10

E78.5

1. Determine any areas of inaccuracy in the CAC identification.

2. Recommend corrections to the code assignment.

Resource

Lee-Eichenwald, S. 2020. Health Information Technologies. Chapter 12 in *Health Information Management: Concepts, Principles, and Practice*, 6th ed. P. Oachs and A. Watters, eds. Chicago: AHIMA.

4.37 Computer-assisted coding roadblock

Competency IV.1RM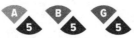

Competency IV.1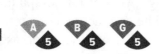

Competency IV.3RM

Coders in your organization have been anxious ever since they heard that computer-assisted coding (CAC) was going to become part of the HIM coding process. They were very worried that their jobs would be lost to a computer program that would do all the coding. After running the test scenario in exercise 4.36, you have a better understanding of a coder's role in the automated process.

1. Explain to your coding staff the importance of coders using CAC as it regards accuracy of codes assigned.

2. Begin a discussion regarding how coders will factor in corrective action regarding CAC.

Resource

Lee-Eichenwald, S. 2020. Health Information Technologies. Chapter 12 in *Health Information Management: Concepts, Principles, and Practice*, 6th ed. P. Oachs and A. Watters, eds. Chicago: AHIMA.

4.38 Evaluate computer-assisted coding systems

Competency IV.2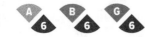

Your organization is in the final stages of selecting a vendor for computer assisted coding. You have narrowed the choices to two vendors and will be conducting conference calls with a current client of each vendor. Formulate a list of questions that will help you assess which product to choose.

Resource

Amatayakul, M. K. 2017. *Health IT and EHRs, Principles and Practice,* 6th ed. Chicago: AHIMA.

4.39 Evaluate MS-DRG and APC groupings

Competency IV.1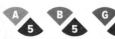

Evaluate the following MS-DRG assignments for accuracy. Defend your answers and provide corrections if necessary.

1. A 12-year-old, intellectually disabled male (IQ=19) was admitted from home with a high fever (105.2) and chills. He had been experiencing a hacking cough for two days prior to admission and was very lethargic. Lab work, sputum culture, rapid flu test, and chest x-ray were performed. Flu test was negative and chest x-ray indicated acute bronchitis. Due to the patient's severely weakened condition and low O_2 levels, he was admitted. After two days in the hospital, where he received IV antibiotics and respiratory treatments for the acute bronchitis, he was much improved and ready for discharge back to his home.

   MS-DRG assigned 203

Admit diagnosis	R50.9
Principal diagnosis	J20.9

2. A 68-year-old female was admitted from skilled nursing with complaints of right flank pain and fever. This developed one day after her last dialysis treatment for CRF. Lab work was drawn, urinalysis performed, and a KUB showed evidence of a renal calculus. The urinalysis indicated a UTI, and the patient was admitted for definitive treatment of the streptococcal B UTI and renal calculus. IV antibiotics were administered, and increased fluids flushed the stone. By the third day, the UTI seemed to be clearing, so the patient was discharged back to skilled care. Her long-standing hypertension was controlled during her admission with Atenolol, which she takes at home.

   MS-DRG assigned 694

Admit diagnosis	R10.9
Principal diagnosis	N20.0
Secondary diagnosis	N39.0
	B95.1
	I10
	N18.9
	Z79.899

3. A 69-year-old male was admitted after arrival in the ED with extreme shortness of breath. He was found to be experiencing an acute exacerbation of his COPD and therefore admitted for treatment. On the second day of his admission, he began complaining of right knee pain. Examination indicated a pyogenic arthritis, and a percutaneous aspiration of the joint was done with appropriate antibiotics started. Two days later, both the patient's respiratory and knee conditions were much improved, and the patient was discharged home.

MS-DRG assigned 192

Admit diagnosis	R06.02
Principal diagnosis	J44.1
Secondary diagnosis	M25.561
Procedure performed	0S9C3ZZ

4. A 72-year-old black male was admitted to the hospital with four-vessel CAD. A diagnostic, left heart catheterization was done and it was determined that the patient needed an immediate bypass procedure. An open, aortocoronary bypass was done of the four vessels with heavy disease utilizing a right leg saphenous vein graft that was harvested percutaneously. The patient's pre-existing diabetes and hypertension were monitored and treated with the same medications as at home, Metformin and Lisinopril respectively. Discharged to home six days after surgery in good condition.

    MS-DRG assigned 236

Admit diagnosis	I25.10
Principal diagnosis	I25.10
Secondary diagnosis	E11.9
	I10
	Z79.84
	Z79.899
Procedure performed	021309W, 06BP3ZZ

Resources

Centers for Disease Control and Prevention. 2019. ICD-10-CM. https://www.cdc.gov/nchs/icd/icd10cm .htm.

Centers for Medicare and Medicaid Services. 2019. ICD-10-PCS. https://www.cms.gov/Medicare /Coding/ICD10/2019-ICD-10-PCS.html.

Chapter 5

Domain V: Health Law and Compliance

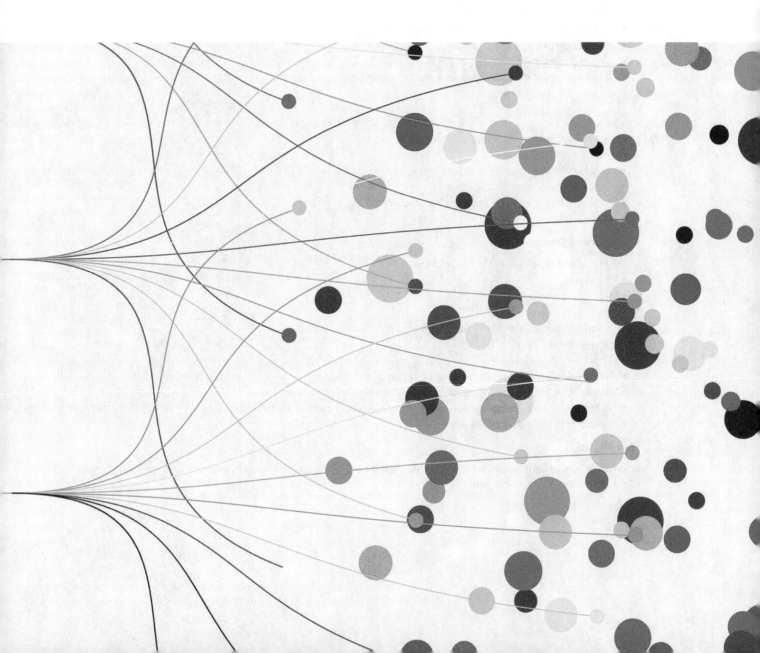

5.0 Notice of privacy practices

Competency V.4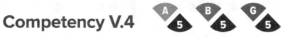

1. Compare the Notice of Privacy Practices (NPP) that follows against the HIPAA and ARRA related elements that must be present in an NPP. Determine if elements are missing and revise the document to include those elements.

2. Why are all the elements necessary?

Your Information. Your Rights. Our Responsibilities.

Your Rights

You have the right to:
- Get a copy of your paper or electronic medical record
- Request confidential communication
- Ask us to limit the information we share
- Get a list of those with whom we've shared your information
- Get a copy of this privacy notice
- Choose someone to act for you
- File a complaint if you believe your privacy rights have been violated

Your Choices

You have some choices in the way that we use and share information as we:
- Tell family and friends about your condition
- Provide disaster relief
- Include you in a hospital directory
- Provide mental health care
- Market our services and sell your information
- Raise funds

Our Uses and Disclosures

We may use and share your information as we:
- Treat you
- Run our organization
- Bill for your services
- Help with public health and safety issues
- Do research
- Comply with the law
- Respond to organ and tissue donation requests
- Work with a medical examiner or funeral director
- Address workers' compensation, law enforcement, and other government requests
- Respond to lawsuits and legal actions

Your Rights

When it comes to your health information, you have certain rights. This section explains your rights and some of our responsibilities to help you.

Get an electronic or paper copy of your medical record

- You can ask to see or get an electronic or paper copy of your medical record and other health information we have about you. Ask us how to do this.
- We will provide a copy or a summary of your health information, usually within 30 days of your request. We may charge a reasonable, cost-based fee.

Request confidential communications

- You can ask us to contact you in a specific way (for example, home or office phone) or to send mail to a different address.
- We will say "yes" to all reasonable requests.

Ask us to limit what we use or share

- You can ask us not to use or share certain health information for treatment, payment, or our operations. We are not required to agree to your request, and we may say "no" if it would affect your care.

Get a list of those with whom we've shared information

- You can ask for a list (accounting) of the times we've shared your health information for six years prior to the date you ask, who we shared it with, and why.
- We will include all the disclosures except for those about treatment, payment, and health care operations, and certain other disclosures (such as any you asked us to make). We'll provide one accounting a year for free but will charge a reasonable, cost-based fee if you ask for another one within 12 months.

Get a copy of this privacy notice

You can ask for a paper copy of this notice at any time, even if you have agreed to receive the notice electronically. We will provide you with a paper copy promptly.

Choose someone to act for you

- If you have given someone medical power of attorney or if someone is your legal guardian, that person can exercise your rights and make choices about your health information.
- We will make sure the person has this authority and can act for you before we take any action.

File a complaint if you feel your rights are violated

- You can complain if you feel we have violated your rights by contacting us using the information on page 1.
- You can file a complaint with the U.S. Department of Health and Human Services Office for Civil Rights by sending a letter to 200 Independence Avenue, S.W., Washington, D.C. 20201, calling 1-877-696-6775, or visiting www.hhs.gov/ocr/privacy/hipaa/complaints/.
- We will not retaliate against you for filing a complaint.

Your Choices

For certain health information, you can tell us your choices about what we share. If you have a clear preference for how we share your information in the situations described below, talk to us. Tell us what you want us to do, and we will follow your instructions.

In these cases, you have both the right and choice to tell us to:

- Share information with your family, close friends, or others involved in your care
- Share information in a disaster relief situation
- Include your information in a hospital directory

If you are not able to tell us your preference, for example if you are unconscious, we may go ahead and share your information if we believe it is in your best interest. We may also share your information when needed to lessen a serious and imminent threat to health or safety.

In these cases, we never share your information unless you give us written permission:

- Marketing purposes
- Sale of your information
- Most sharing of psychotherapy notes

In the case of fundraising:

- We may contact you for fundraising efforts, but you can tell us not to contact you again.

Our Uses and Disclosures

How do we typically use or share your health information?

We typically use or share your health information in the following ways.

Treat you

We can use your health information and share it with other professionals who are treating you.
Example: A doctor treating you for an injury asks another doctor about your overall health condition.

Run our organization

We can use and share your health information to run our practice, improve your care, and contact you when necessary.
Example: We use health information about you to manage your treatment and services.

Bill for your services

We can use and share your health information to bill and get payment from health plans or other entities.
Example: We give information about you to your health insurance plan so it will pay for your services.

How else can we use or share your health information?

We are allowed or required to share your information in other ways – usually in ways that contribute to the public good, such as public health and research. We have to meet many conditions in the law before we can share your information for these purposes. For more information see: www.hhs.gov/ocr/privacy/hipaa/understanding/consumers/index.html.

Help with public health and safety issues

We can share health information about you for certain situations such as:

- Preventing disease
- Helping with product recalls
- Reporting adverse reactions to medications
- Reporting suspected abuse, neglect, or domestic violence
- Preventing or reducing a serious threat to anyone's health or safety

Do research

We can use or share your information for health research.

Comply with the law

We will share information about you if state or federal laws require it, including with the Department of Health and Human Services if it wants to see that we're complying with federal privacy law.

Respond to organ and tissue donation requests

We can share health information about you with organ procurement organizations.

Work with a medical examiner or funeral director

We can share health information with a coroner, medical examiner, or funeral director when an individual dies.

Address workers' compensation, law enforcement, and other government requests

We can use or share health information about you:

- For workers' compensation claims
- For law enforcement purposes or with a law enforcement official
- With health oversight agencies for activities authorized by law
- For special government functions such as military, national security, and presidential protective services

Respond to lawsuits and legal actions

We can share health information about you in response to a court or administrative order, or in response to a subpoena.

Our Responsibilities

- We are required by law to maintain the privacy and security of your protected health information.
- We will let you know promptly if a breach occurs that may have compromised the privacy or security of your information.
- We must follow the duties and privacy practices described in this notice and give you a copy of it.
- We will not use or share your information other than as described here unless you tell us we can in writing. If you tell us we can, you may change your mind at any time. Let us know in writing if you change your mind.

For more information see: www.hhs.gov/ocr/privacy/hipaa/understanding/consumers/noticepp.html.

Changes to the Terms of this Notice

We can change the terms of this notice, and the changes will apply to all information we have about you. The new notice will be available upon request, in our office, and on our web site.

Source: HHS 2013.

Resources

Department of Health and Human Services (HHS). 2013. Model Notices of Privacy Practices. http://www.hhs.gov/ocr/privacy/hipaa/modelnotices.html.

Rinehart-Thompson, L.A. 2017. HIPAA Privacy Rule: Part 1. Chapter 10 in *Fundamentals of Law for Health Informatics and Information Management*, 3rd ed. M.S. Brodnik, L. A. Rinehart-Thompson, and R. B. Reynolds, eds. Chicago: AHIMA.

5.1 Joint Commission—Do Not Use abbreviations I

Competency V.1

Competency V.4

Visit the Joint Commission website to obtain the Joint Commission's Do Not Use Abbreviation (DNUA) list (Joint Commission 2019). Examine the sample transcription reports and compare them with the DNUA list. Determine any error(s) found that conflict with the DNUA list and recommend the necessary corrections.

Report 1

Procedure:	Trigger Point Injection
Anesthesia:	Local and MAC
Complications:	None

Procedure: The 48-year-old white female was brought to the procedure suite. After reviewing the risks, benefits, and alternatives to the procedure, she decided to procedure with the trigger point injection. Her upper back was sterilely prepped. I isolated the muscle in spasm and used a 25-gauge 5-inch needle to perform an aspiration of the area, which was negative. Then 4.0 cc of Marcaine .5 percent was injected into three trigger points. She tolerated the procedure very well.

Report 2

Procedure:	Right prepatellar bursal injection
Anesthesia:	MAC
Complications:	None

This 57-year-old black male has acute prepatellar bursitis. The right knee is swollen and warm to the touch. He has had similar symptoms in the past, responded well to Aristospan injection, and is here today for an injection.

I reviewed the risks, benefits, and alternatives to the procedure with the patient, who expressed his understanding and agreed to proceed with the injection. MAC sedation was initiated and I prepped the knee with a sterile alcohol wipe. I then injected 20.0 mg of Aristospan into the right prepatellar bursa. No complications from the injection were noted. Discharge after criteria met. Instructed patient it was okay to continue his Novolog 100 U before each meal for his type I diabetes.

Resources

Rinehart-Thompson, L. A. 2017. Legal Health Record: Maintenance, Content, Documentation, and Disposition. Chapter 9 in *Fundamentals of Law for Health Informatics and Information Management*, 3rd ed. M. S. Brodnik, L. A. Rinehart-Thompson, and R. B. Reynolds. Chicago: AHIMA.

Joint Commission. 2019. Facts about the Official "Do Not Use" List of Abbreviations. https://www.jointcommission.org/facts_about_do_not_use_list/.

Shaw, P. L. and D. Carter. 2019. Building a Safe Medication Management System. Chapter 12 in *Quality and Performance Improvement in Healthcare: Theory, Practice, and Management,* 7th ed. Chicago: AHIMA.

5.2 Joint Commission—Do Not Use abbreviations II

Competency V.2

Competency V.4

As the HIM director for Riverdale Medical Center, you co-chair the medical records committee with Dr. Taylor, an internal medicine doctor. Dr. Taylor has presented an agenda item for the next meeting to discuss additions to Riverdale's do-not-use abbreviation list. She is proposing the addition of two new abbreviations to the current list mandated by the Joint Commission. You are against adding any more abbreviations to the current list. Defend your position by creating bullet points of the key reasons for leaving the list as is. Provide at least three reasons.

Resources

Joint Commission. 2019. Facts about the Official "Do Not Use" List of Abbreviations. http://www .jointcommission.org/facts_about_do_not_use_list/.

Rinehart-Thompson, L. A. 2017. Legal Health Record: Maintenance, Content, Documentation, and Disposition. Chapter 9 in *Fundamentals of Law for Health Informatics and Information Management*, 3rd ed. M. S. Brodnik, L. A. Rinehart-Thompson, and R. B. Reynolds. Chicago: AHIMA.

B

G

5.3 Present on admission

A

B

G

Competency V.3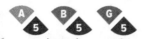

You have just taken a job as an inpatient coder at Pine Valley Community Hospital, a critical access hospital (CAH), after previously working at a large teaching facility in the same role. During your training at PVCH, you are surprised that the trainer stated that you do not have to assign the present on admission (POA) status on inpatient discharges. You decide to research this practice. After research, prove the trainer's statement is correct. Provide reasons and at least two Centers for Medicare and Medicaid references used in your research.

Resources

Centers for Medicare and Medicaid Services (CMS). 2019a. Hospital-Acquired Conditions (Present on Admission Indicator) Affected Hospitals. https://www.cms.gov/Medicare/Medicare-Fee-for-Service -Payment/HospitalAcqCond/AffectedHospitals.html.

Centers for Medicare and Medicaid Services (CMS). 2019b. Medicare Learning Network: Critical Access Hospitals. https://www.cms.gov/Outreach-and-Education/Medicare-Learning-Network-MLN /MLNProducts/downloads/critaccesshospfctsht.pdf.

5.4 Present on admission analysis

Competency V.3 A 5 B 5 G 5

1. Determine the present on admission (POA) status for the following scenarios.
    a. A newborn suffers a dislocated shoulder during delivery. What is the POA status for the shoulder dislocation?
    b. A child fell from the jungle gym at the school playground and was taken to the emergency room for treatment since she was complaining of pain in her elbow. She was diagnosed with a supracondylar fracture of the humerus and was taken directly to the operating room. Immediately after surgery, she experienced severe postoperative nausea and vomiting and was then admitted as an inpatient for rehydration. Assign the POA status for the:

    -   Supracondylar fracture
    -   Post-op nausea and vomiting
    -   Fall from jungle gym

2. Determine if the following POA status assignments are correct. If the assigned POA is not correct, indicate what change should be made to correct the assignment.
    a. Physician notes genetic susceptibility for breast malignancy in patient's record

    Code assigned was Z15.01   POA assigned was Y

    b. Patient admitted with chest pain. In the progress note of the second day, the physician states the patient had a mild NSTEMI (non-ST elevation myocardial infarction).

    Code assigned was I21.4   POA assigned was N

    c. Three days after hip replacement surgery, the physician documents "Rule out pneumonia" in a progress note after noting fever and cough upon examination. At discharge, the physician documents pneumonia as one of the discharge diagnoses.

    Code assigned was J18.9   POA assigned was Y

Resource

Optum360. 2019. Present on Admission Reporting Guidelines. Appendix I in *ICD-10-CM Expert for Hospitals*. Salt Lake City: Optum.

5.5 Tracer methodology

Competency V.2

A new director of quality at the organization where you are the health information management (HIM) director wants to meet to discuss your role in Joint Commission preparation specifically as it relates to tracer methodology. You consider the role that HIM has had on tracer methodology preparation. Determine at least three ways that HIM has assisted in the tracer process as you prepare for the upcoming meeting.

Resources

HCPro. 2004 (January). *HIM-HIPAA Insider*. Preparing for Tracer Methodology. http://www.hcpro.com /HIM-37036-865/Preparing-for-Tracer-Methodology.html.

Shaw, P. L. and D. Carter. 2019. *Quality and Performance Improvement in Healthcare, A Tool for Programmed Learning,* 7th ed. Chicago: AHIMA.

5.6 Delinquent medical records

Competency V.2

When you came on board as HIM director, an issue needing immediate attention was the high delinquency rate of medical record completion. In fact, at the last The Joint Commission survey, the organization received a zero (0) for insufficient compliance with this standard.

The organization's current practice is that a letter is sent to physicians once charts have become delinquent at 30 days post-discharge. Follow-up letters continue weekly, and if charts were not completed, the previous director would call the physician office. Strategize solutions to the high delinquency rate.

1. Recommend a minimum of four options that could be implemented easily and have a positive impact on the record completion process.

2. Note three options that will take longer to implement and assess the pros and cons of implementing those options.

Resources

Medical Staff Briefing. 2007 (July). Knock out Medical Record Delinquencies. http://healthleadersmedia.com/content/HOM-90847/Knock-out-medical-record-delinquencies.html.

Reynolds, R. and A. Morey. 2020. Health Record Content and Documentation. Chapter 4 in *Health Information Management: Concepts, Principles, and Practice*, 6th ed. P. Oachs and A. Watters, eds. Chicago: AHIMA.

A

B

5.7 Fraud and abuse focus

Competency V.3

Although you are new to your role as revenue cycle manager, you are nonetheless surprised to learn that there is no formal process in place for isolating potential areas of compliance concern. You recognize that this would be generated from a focused approach for internal or external auditing, leading to identification of coding compliance concerns and opportunities for coder education. Recommend to the coding supervisor a minimum of four best practices for determining focus areas for auditing and monitoring of coding compliance.

Resources

D'Amato, C. and G. I. Kelley. 2008. Benchmarking Coding Quality. http://campus.ahima.org /audio/2008/RB072408.pdf.

Hunt, T. J. and K. Kirk. 2020. Clinical Documentation Improvement and Coding Compliance. Chapter 9 in *Health Information Management: Concepts, Principles, and Practice*, 6th ed. P. Oachs and A. Watters, eds. Chicago: AHIMA.

5.8 Stark anti-kickback

Competency V.3

You are the new practice manager for Meadow Pediatric Care, a pediatric primary care group owned by Dr. Charles Greene, that serves a large Medicaid population. As you review policies, you find that *all* referrals for speech-language pathology services are made to Children's Speech and Language Services of Valley View (CSLSVV), which is one of three area businesses that supply those services to children. As it happens, your son has had services from the CSLSVV, and you know that business is owned by Dr. Greene's sister, Dr. Sherry Watt.

1. What could this discovery mean for Dr. Thomas? Apply the appropriate federal statute.

2. Upon further investigation, you find that a monthly deposit is being made from CSLSVV into the pediatric groups account. What could be inferred from this transaction and what federal statute would apply?

3. Could the term "safe harbor" have any relevance in this scenario? Justify your answer.

Resources

Bowman, S. 2017. Corporate Compliance. Chapter 18 in *Fundamentals of Law for Health Informatics and Information Management,* 3rd ed. M. S. Brodnik, L. A. Rinehart-Thompson, and R. B. Reynolds, eds. Chicago: AHIMA.

Edelstein, S. A. 2007. Implementing the new Stark Law exceptions and anti-kickback safe harbors for electronic prescribing and electronic health records. AHIMA's 79th National Convention and Exhibit Proceedings. Philadelphia, PA.

5.9 Whistleblower

Competency V.3

Competency V.4

As an inpatient coder, you have been instructed by your coding supervisor to code all debridements as excisional. You are not comfortable with this practice and tried to discuss it with her, but she stated that you were to follow her instructions and not issue queries. You went to the HIM director, who only half-listened to your concerns, saying that the coding supervisor must have a good reason for the instruction. The other coders are following her instructions without question.

You are reluctant to get into trouble for not following the instructions and equally worried that the coding supervisor will retaliate against you in some manner if you report this practice.

1. Assess and provide a minimum of three options you have in this situation.

2. Appraise the impact of the False Claims Act as it relates to this situation.

Resource

Bowman, S. 2017. Corporate Compliance. Chapter 18 in *Fundamentals of Law for Health Informatics and Information Management*, 3rd ed. M. S. Brodnik, L. A. Rinehart-Thompson, and R. B. Reynolds, eds. Chicago: AHIMA.

5.10 Bilateral reporting

Competency V.2

A recent audit of hospital accounts with bilateral cataract procedures coded showed the following:

35 accounts coded	66984-RT Unit of service 1
	66984-LT Unit of service 1
172 accounts coded	66984-50 Unit of service 1
7 accounts coded	66984 Unit of service 1
	66984-50 Unit of service 1
2 accounts coded	66984 Unit of service 2

Develop a coding procedure for bilateral cataract procedures that will comply with the National Correct Coding Initiative.

Resources

Centers for Medicare and Medicaid Services. 2019. *NCCI Policy Manual for Medicare Services.* https://www.cms.gov/Medicare/Coding/NationalCorrectCodInitEd/index.html?redirect= /NationalCorrectCodInitEd/.

Hazelwood, A. 2020. Reimbursement Methodologies. Chapter 7 in *Health Information Management: Concepts, Principles, and Practice*, 6th ed. P. Oachs and A. Watters, eds. Chicago: AHIMA.

5.11 Compliance policy

Competency V.2

As the new coding manager at St. Stephen's Hospital, you are surprised to learn there is no coding compliance plan in place. Begin drafting at least six policies and procedures that would be appropriate in a coding compliance plan. Elaborate on the importance of including these proposals in the coding compliance plan.

Resources

Hunt, T. J. and K. Kirk. 2020. Clinical Documentation Improvement and Coding Compliance. Chapter 9 in *Health Information Management: Concepts, Principles, and Practice*, 6th ed. P. Oachs and A. Watters, eds. Chicago: AHIMA.

Prophet, S. 1998. Coding compliance: practical strategies for success. *Journal of AHIMA* 69(1):50–61.

5.12 Fraud trend analysis

Competency V.3

In your role as revenue cycle manager, you are looking at the data below to determine how your organization's coding of COPD as a principal diagnosis compares with other local facilities as well as on the state and national levels.

1. Create tables to illustrate the comparison of three hospitals, with the state and national percentages for the distribution of MS-DRGs 190-192 using the data below.

2. Predict how each hospital might react to analysis of these tables.

3. Hospital X represents your facility's information. Do those results raise any concerns for you?

MS-DRG 190 discharges

Hospital X	38
Hospital Y	112
Hospital Z	89
State	8,300
Nation	315,400

MS-DRG 191 discharges

Hospital X	23
Hospital Y	104
Hospital Z	31
State	7,912
Nation	290,565

MS-DRG 192 discharges

Hospital X	18
Hospital Y	67
Hospital Z	17
State	2,214
Nation	93,214

Resources

Casto, A. B. 2018. Medicare-Medicaid Prospective Payment Systems for Inpatients. Chapter 6 in *Principles of Healthcare Reimbursement*, 6th ed. Chicago: AHIMA.

Hunt, T. J. and K. Kirk. 2020. Reimbursement Methodologies. Chapter 7 in *Health Information Management: Concepts, Principles, and Practice*, 6th ed. Chicago: AHIMA.

McNeill, M. H. 2020. Healthcare Statistics. Chapter 14 in *Health Information Management Technology: An Applied Approach*, 6th ed. N. B. Sayles and L. Gordon, eds. Chicago: AHIMA.

5.13 Patient-centered medical home I

Competency V.4

You have a friend who works as a medical assistant for a local primary care practice. She recently mentioned that the group is planning to transition to a patient-centered medical home model (PCMH) and are looking for someone with a strong background in health information management (HIM) to assist in the transition. She knows that you hold an RHIT certification and thought you might be interested.

You are intrigued by her comments and wonder if you have the necessary qualifications and background to become part of that team. Your job, which you obtained upon graduation a year ago, has been in information systems at a small local hospital. Your current project is implementing a new denials management tool, which you are managing from start to finish.

Investigate this PCMH model of primary care and assess the qualifications and background that an HIM professional could bring to that project. Determine areas where your qualifications and background may be weak.

Resources

Casto, A. B. 2018. Value-Based Purchasing. Chapter 10 in *Principles of Healthcare Reimbursement*, 6th ed. Chicago: AHIMA.

Dimick, C. 2008. Home Sweet Medical Home: Can a New Care Model Save Family Medicine? *Journal of AHIMA* 79(8):24–28.

5.14 Patient-centered medical home II

Competency V.4

After reviewing the information from case 5.13 on patient-centered medical homes (PCMH), you decide to apply for the HIM position now available at that primary care practice. Draft responses to the following questions as you prepare for your upcoming interview.

1. What do you know about the reimbursement process for PCMHs? How does it compare to capitation?

2. What are some ways that the PCMH model could save healthcare dollars?

Resources

Casto, A. B. 2018. Value-Based Purchasing. Chapter 10 in *Principles of Healthcare Reimbursement,* 6th ed. Chicago: AHIMA.

Dimick, C. 2008. Home Sweet Medical Home: Can a New Care Model Save Family Medicine? *Journal of AHIMA* 79(8):24–28.

5.15 Videotaping policy

Competency V.2

Pine Valley Community Hospital, a critical access hospital, is considering participation in an educational project for medical students. Under the proposal, they will videotape the events of the emergency department 24/7 for one week. In your role as HIM director, you have been asked to identify and interpret any Joint Commission standards that might impact such an agreement and report back to the administration.

a. Assess and interpret any Joint Commission information on the topic of videotaping.

b. Formulate a policy that would ensure compliance with the intent of the standard.

Resources

LeBlanc, M. M. 2020. Human Resources Management. Chapter 22 in *Health Information Management: Concepts, Principles, and Practice*, 6th ed. P. Oachs and A. Watters, eds. Chicago: AHIMA.

The Joint Commission. n.d.a. Videotaping in a critical access hospital. *Standards Interpretation*. Accessed 29 March 2019. https://www.jointcommission.org/standards_information/jcfaqdetails.aspx?StandardsFAQId=834&StandardsFAQChapterId=31&ProgramId=0&ChapterId=0&IsFeatured=False&IsNew=False&Keyword=videotaping.

The Joint Commission. n.d.b. Rights and Responsibilities of the Individual (RI) (Critical Access Hospitals / Critical Access Hospitals): Videotaping or Filming – Consent Not Provided by Patient's Portion. *Standards FAQ Details*. Accessed 12 May 2019. https://www.jointcommission.org/standards_information/jcfaqdetails.aspx?StandardsFAQId=833&StandardsFAQChapterId=31&ProgramId=0&ChapterId=0&IsFeatured=False&IsNew=False&Keyword=videotaping.

The Joint Commission. n.d.c. Rights and Responsibilities of the Individual (RI) (Critical Access Hospitals / Critical Access Hospitals): Videotaping or Filming - Consent Not Provided. *Standards FAQ Details*. Accessed 12 May 2019. https://www.jointcommission.org/standards_information/jcfaqdetails.aspx?StandardsFAQId=832&StandardsFAQChapterId=31&ProgramId=0&ChapterId=0&IsFeatured=False&IsNew=False&Keyword=videotaping.

The Joint Commission. n.d.d. Rights and Responsibilities of the Individual (RI) (Critical Access Hospitals / Critical Access Hospitals): Videotaping or Filming in the Emergency Room - Consent. Standards FAQ Details. Accessed 12 May 2019. https://www.jointcommission.org/standards_information/jcfaqdetails.aspx?StandardsFAQId=835&StandardsFAQChapterId=31&ProgramId=0&ChapterId=0&IsFeatured=False&IsNew=False&Keyword=videotaping.

5.16 Legal terminology I

Competency V.1

Mrs. Barbara White was admitted to Richmond Medical Center for hip replacement surgery. Preoperatively, she was administered a prophylactic medication to reduce postoperative gastrointestinal complications as part of surgeon Dr. Gilchrist's, standing orders. Unfortunately, Mrs. White had an allergy to the medication, which was listed in her medical record but went unnoticed by staff. Once the error was recognized, Benadryl was given to counteract the original medication, but that caused a steep drop in her blood pressure, which led to a stroke. Mrs. White suffered dysphasia and hemiplegia, which continue to this day.

Mrs. White sued Dr. Gilchrist and the nursing staff for damages as a result of the injuries she sustained. Her attorney, Monique LeClair, recognized the need to move quickly to preserve the documentation related to the case.

1. Based on that necessity, the attorney's first step should be to ask the court for what?

2. Demonstrate why that is a necessary step in this proceeding.

Next, knowing that RMC's medical records were hybrid, Ms. LeClair needed access to the electronic documents which were part of her patient's record along with any e-mails that may have been pertinent to the case.

Documents were then exchanged between the various lawyers and members of the hospital staff gave pretrial oral testimony. Upon reviewing documents from the hospital, Ms. LeClair's team found a metadata discrepancy on an e-form used to document the patient's vital signs. The attorney had the court issue an order for nurse responsible for the documentation to appear at the trial. Based on the nurse's statement at trial that the document had been altered to reflect constant vital sign monitoring with no substantial change, the deciders of fact supported Mrs. White and awarded 4.3 million dollars in damages.

3. Identify the appropriate healthcare legal terminology for the items from the scenario.
   a. Mrs. Barbara White
   b. Dr. Gilchrist and Richmond Medical Center
   c. Court issued order requiring the nurse to appear at the trial
   d. Deciders of fact
   e. Pretrial exchange of documents between lawyers
   f. Pretrial oral testimony
   g. Electronic documents
   h. Statement at trial

Resources

Klaver, J. C. 2017. Evidence. Chapter 5 in *Fundamentals of Law for Health Informatics and Information Management,* 3rd ed. M. S. Brodnik, L. A. Rinehart-Thompson, and R. B. Reynolds, eds. Chicago: AHIMA.

Rinehart-Thompson, L. A. 2017. Legal Proceedings. Chapter 4 in *Fundamentals of Law for Health Informatics and Information Management,* 3rd ed. M. S. Brodnik, L. A. Rinehart-Thompson, and R. B. Reynolds, eds. Chicago: AHIMA.

5.17 Healthcare laws and HIM

Competency V.1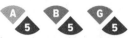

As an HIM professional at a behavioral health facility, you have been asked to be a panel member on the topic of privacy and security for a state HIM association meeting. The facilitator of the event has asked that you choose three laws, regulations, or events that pertain to privacy and security, especially as they relate to behavioral health patient information, to share with the attendees. Prepare a brief synopsis of their relevance to privacy and security and interpret their relationship to each other in that regard.

Resources

Brodnik, M. S.2017. Access, Use, and Disclosure and Release of Health Information. Chapter 15 in *Fundamentals of Law for Health Informatics and Information Management,* 3rd ed. M. S. Brodnik, L. A. Rinehart-Thompson, and R. B. Reynolds, eds. Chicago: AHIMA.

Reynolds, R. B. and M. S. Brodnik. 2017. The HIPAA Security Rule. Chapter 12 in *Fundamentals of Law for Health Informatics and Information Management,* 3rd ed. M. S. Brodnik, L. A. Rinehart-Thompson, and R. B. Reynolds, eds. Chicago: AHIMA.

Rinehart-Thompson, L. A. 2017a. The HIPAA Privacy Rule: Part 1. Chapter 10 in *Fundamentals of Law for Health Informatics and Information Management,* 3rd ed. M. S. Brodnik, L. A. Rinehart-Thompson, and R. B. Reynolds, eds. Chicago: AHIMA.

Rinehart-Thompson, L. A. 2017b. The HIPAA Privacy Rule: Part II. Chapter 11 in *Fundamentals of Law for Health Informatics and Information Management,* 3rd ed. M. S. Brodnik, L. A. Rinehart-Thompson, and R. B. Reynolds, eds. Chicago: AHIMA.

5.18 Subpoena preparation

Competency V.2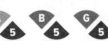

As the HIM director, you have been served with a subpoena to produce records for an upcoming court case. Your release of information clerk is new, and when you direct her to the procedure to follow for preparing records in response to a subpoena, you find there is not one. Select the steps to include in the procedure and outline them.

Resources

Demster, B., A. K. Dinh, S. Emery, E. R. Gorton, and J. R. Lantis, Jr. 2012. Management Practices for the Release of Information. *Journal of AHIMA* 83(2).

Rinehart-Thompson, L. A. 2017. Legal Proceedings. Chapter 4 in *Fundamentals of Law for Health Informatics and Information Management,* 3rd ed. M. S. Brodnik, L. A. Rinehart-Thompson, and R. B. Reynolds, eds. Chicago: AHIMA.

5.19 Legal document conundrum

A

Competency V.1 A 3

Correctly identify the appropriate legal document required for each scenario below.

1. After serious consideration, Harry has decided to undergo a new and extremely delicate heart procedure. At 56, his hypertrophic cardiomyopathy has required him to adopt a sedentary lifestyle. Medication no longer manages his disease, so surgery is the option of last resort. After careful consideration, Harry has decided that if he should suffer a cardiac or respiratory arrest, he does not want any cardiopulmonary resuscitation. What specific legal document should Harry complete and share with his healthcare providers?

2. Prior to Harry's heart surgery, his physician will discuss Harry's diagnosis and the procedure in detail. He will share any alternatives to the surgery, outline the benefits of the procedure, and discuss the risks associated with the procedure. Harry will have the opportunity to ask any questions he may have regarding the surgery. The physician will then complete what legal document that certifies that the patient has been made aware of this information?

3. Early onset familial Alzheimer's disease runs in Ruth's family. Her mother had the disease, and Ruth has just had genetic testing, which indicates that she will have the disease as well. After her initial shock, Ruth has decided to be proactive with her healthcare and, to that end, has decided to appoint her daughter to make healthcare decisions for her once she is unable to make them for herself. Ruth needs to complete what legal document to ensure that her daughter is legally empowered to make those decisions?

4. Martha has learned that she has metastatic breast cancer. Her physicians have indicated that she will need a mastectomy along with chemotherapy and radiation therapy. She recognizes that there could be many obstacles and setbacks as she fights this disease and that there could come a time that she would be unable to make her own decisions. To that end, Martha has decided to complete a legal document outlining her wishes for treatment if she is ever unable to communicate them for herself. What legal document should Martha complete?

5. George is an eighty-year-old man in relatively good health. However, he sees many of his friends dealing with healthcare issues and how, sometimes, families bicker over the healthcare decisions of a loved one who is incapacitated. George would like to be confident that no issues like that would arise in the event of a decline in his mental function, so he is going to issue what type of legal document(s) that will be effective in the event he becomes incapacitated?

Resource

Klaver, J. C. 2017. Consent to Treatment. Chapter 8 in *Fundamentals of Law for Health Informatics and Information Management*, 3rd ed. M. S. Brodnik, L. A. Rinehart-Thompson, R. B. Reynolds, eds. Chicago: AHIMA.

5.20 Legal health record maintenance

Competency V.1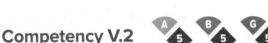

Competency V.2

Judge each scenario that follows to determine if the documentation practice presented would be legally defensible, meaning does it meet regulatory, accreditation, legal, and professional practice standards? Defend your answer.

1. Discharge summary dictated on 11/24/19 for a patient discharged on 9/30/19

2. Process whereby emergency department reports that are transcribed are considered approved and signed if no corrections are made to the transcription within 48 hours of posting

3. A faxed order and signature for a patient to receive physical therapy

4. The following order with a rubber-stamped signature:
   Turn patient every 2 hours to prevent decubitus ulcers.
       Dr. Timothy Reynolds 12/2/19 11:15 a.m.

5. The correction shown here:
   Administer two units of ~~fresh frozen plasma~~. ERROR –wrong blood product TR 12/18/19, 5:27 p.m.
       Dr. Timothy Reynolds 12/18/19 5:25 p.m.
   Administer two units of packed red cells.
       Dr. Timothy Reynolds 12/18/19 5:30 p.m.

6. In a patient's EHR for his last inpatient admission, a coder notices that the operative report is located under the discharge summary tab and brings it to your attention. You have it moved to the correct location within the account without annotation.

7. Nursing documentation for 10/31/19:
       3:00 p.m.–11:00 p.m. Administered dose of antibiotic. Walked patient in hallway. Sat patient up in chair. Performed vitals. Assisted patient back to bed. Checked on patient-resting comfortably, no pain. Walked patient in hallway and assisted to bathroom. Checked vitals. Administered antibiotic and pain medication.

8. Physician order:
   Give Lotensin 20mg. daily
   ─────── *10/26/19 2:55p.m.*

9. A physician copies and pastes his progress note from two days ago into his most current note, adding a brief comment that there is no change in the patient's condition.

Progress note 11/4/19
Patient showing improvement in breathing. Responding well to antibiotic. Able to get out of bed and move around with assistance. Performed a bedside debridement of a lower leg ulcer, excisional, subcutaneous.

Progress note 11/6/19

Patient showing improvement in breathing. Responding well to antibiotic. Able to get out of bed and move around with assistance. Performed a bedside debridement of a lower leg ulcer, excisional, subcutaneous.

No change. Continued improvement.

10. An organization has a policy for record retention that states hard copies are kept for seven years. In 2019, records purged for destruction included the following list:

MR #	YEAR
0015698	2011
0051482	2010
0742412	2009
0089364	2010
0009332	2011
0041127	2009
0065435	2012
0126525	2008
0039254	2009
0001153	2011
0248761	2010
0044879	2005
0964578	2010
0676766	2011
0037526	2009

Resources

AHIMA e-HIM Work Group on Maintaining the Legal EHR. 2005. Update: Maintaining a Legally Sound Health Record—Paper and Electronic. *Journal of AHIMA* 76(10):64A-L.

Reynolds, R. and A. Morey. 2020. Health Record Content and Documentation. Chapter 4 in *Health Information Management: Concepts, Principles, and Practice*, 6th ed. P. Oachs and A. Watters, eds. Chicago: AHIMA.

Rinehart-Thompson, L. A. 2017. Legal Health Record: Maintenance, Content, Documentation, and Disposition. Chapter 9 in *Fundamentals of Law for Health Informatics and Information Management*, 3rd ed. M. S. Brodnik, L. A. Rinehart-Thompson, R. B. Reynolds, eds. Chicago: AHIMA.

5.21 Legal terminology II

Competency V.1

Nellie is a 24-year-old waitress at Pete's Diner. She was in her primary care doctor's office for an HPV vaccine, and several regulars from the diner were also there for appointments. When it was Nellie's turn to be seen, the medical assistant said to Nellie as she escorted her to the treatment room, "You're here for the HIV injection, right?" Two of Nellie's regular customers were walking to the front desk and overheard the medical assistant's comments. Nellie corrected the medical assistant, but by that time they were in the treatment room. When Nellie was finished at the doctor's office, she went to work, where she was greeted by Pete, who told her she was fired. He had heard about the HIV comment from customers and could not afford to lose business because his regular customers were upset.

1. Decide which type of character defamation was portrayed in this scenario.

2. Consider the defenses that might be used on behalf of the medical assistant. Provide an opinion on whether any or all of the defenses will absolve the medical assistant of liability and support your position.

Resource

Rinehart-Thompson, L. A. 2017. Tort Law. Chapter 6 in *Fundamentals of Law for Health Informatics and Information Management,* 3rd ed. M. S. Brodnick, L. A. Rinehart-Thompson, and R. B. Reynolds, eds. Chicago: AHIMA.

5.22 Subpoenas and documentation

Competency V.2

While conducting the preparation of a record in response to a subpoena received on 12/10/18, you realize that there is a potential legal issue with the discharge summary. Give your opinion about the discharge summary that follows and what issue(s) it presents.

PATIENT: Jane Johnson **MR#:** 1026336

DISCHARGE DATE: 9/24/18 **DISCHARGE DIAGNOSIS:** Infection right hip prosthesis

ADDITIONAL DISCHARGE DIAGNOSES:

1. Hypertension
2. Type II diabetes
3. Tobacco use
4. Chronic renal failure
5. Restless leg syndrome

REASON FOR ADMISSION: 74-year-old white female admitted with an infected right hip prosthesis. The patient presented to my office with low-grade fever, and slight redness, accompanied by warmth over the previous incision. She directly admitted to the hospital.

HOSPITAL COURSE: The patient was admitted on 9/19/18 and was immediately started on IV antibiotics. She was encouraged to keep the extremity elevated. A wound culture was taken and returned as MRSA. I then changed the antibiotic to Vancomycin. Daily wound care was provided. During the stay, the patient's smoking was addressed, and I indicated that continued smoking will delay healing and strongly urged the patient to quit smoking. On day one, the patient's hypertension was extremely elevated at 165-110. Cardene was administered and the blood pressure responded, eventually maintaining at 130-90. Edema of her lower extremities was reported and consult obtained. Concern was that her chronic hepatitis C was causing the edema, but consultant felt it was secondary to chronic venous stasis. The patient's progress was slow but steady. Compression was added to the treatment and by 09/24/18 her wound had only minimal redness and swelling was down with compression. The patient was discharged home to self care.

DISCHARGE INSTRUCTIONS: The patient was discharged on doxycycline 100 mg p.o. b.i.d. ×10 days along with pain medication of OxyContin. She was instructed how to perform daily wound care with followup in my office in two weeks.

DISCHARGE CONDITION: Stable.

Dr. Stephen Williams

Dr. Stephen Williams
Dictated: 12/3/18
Electronically signed: 12/4/18

Resources

Reynolds, R. and A. Morey. 2020. Health Record Content and Documentation. Chapter 4 in *Health Information Management: Concepts, Principles, and Practice*, 6th ed. P. Oachs and A. Watters, eds. Chicago: AHIMA.

Rinehart-Thompson, L. A. 2017. Legal Health Record: Maintenance, Content, Documentation, and Disposition. Chapter 9 in *Fundamentals of Law for Health Informatics and Information Management*, 3rd ed. M. S. Brodnik, L. A. Rinehart-Thompson, and R. B. Reynolds, eds. Chicago: AHIMA.

5.23 Subpoenas and testifying

Competency V.2

Assume that you have now been called to testify regarding the record discussed in 5.22. The plaintiff's counsel suspect that the discharge summary presented is not the original document. As the HIM director, you are questioned about the version management process at your organization. Distinguish between draft (pending) and finalized status, and indicate the status of the discharge summary. Provide your opinion on whether or not this information will satisfy plaintiff's counsel.

Reference

Rinehart-Thompson, L. A. 2017. Legal Health Record: Maintenance, Content, Documentation, and Disposition. Chapter 9 in *Fundamentals of Law for Health Informatics and Information Management*, 3rd ed. M. S. Brodnik, L. A. Rinehart-Thompson, and R. B. Reynolds, eds. Chicago: AHIMA.

5.24 Legal terminology III

Competency V.1

Susan R. went to the Reynolds Medical Imaging Pavilion for her first mammogram. She signed in, presented her information and order, and then took a seat in the waiting room. 10 minutes later, the technician called for Susan and she went back to the room. She was told to remove her blouse and bra, put on the gown with the opening in the front, and then lie on the table face down. Slightly confused but thinking this must be a new method for mammograms, she did as she was told. Five minutes later, a physician came into the room and performed a breast biopsy on her.

The patient was shocked when the procedure began and attempted to explain to the physician that there was a mistake, but the physician proceeded with the biopsy. Afterwards, it was determined that Susan B. was the patient who was scheduled for a biopsy, not Susan R. Only Susan B. signed a consent form for the biopsy.

Susan R. began having nightmares after the procedure. This was accompanied by extreme anxiety when anyone came too close to her. After a conversation with her husband, she contacted a lawyer to initiate a lawsuit.

Apply the concept of torts to this scenario and distinguish which type(s) of tort is(are) depicted. Provide support for your answer.

Resource

Rinehart-Thompson, L. A. 2017. Tort Law. Chapter 6 in *Fundamentals of Law for Health Informatics and Information Management*, 3rd ed. M. S. Brodnik, L. A. Rinehart-Thompson, and R. B. Reynolds, eds. Chicago: AHIMA.

5.25 Consent

Competency V.1

Last week, a 26-year-old, 36-week pregnant female showed up at the emergency department. As she was walking into the building alone, she grabbed her head and fell to the ground. Staff rushed her to the emergency department, where it was discovered that she had accelerated hypertension of 225/140. She suffered a seizure, lapsing into a coma, and severe stroke was diagnosed. Vital signs were not able to be stabilized and the decision was made to perform an emergency c-section to save the baby. Shortly after the surgery, the woman died as a result of the stroke. Staff had been unable to contact a family member as the woman did not have a purse, wallet, or phone on her person when she came in.

1. What type(s) of consent can be applied to this scenario?

2. How might the lack of consent(s) obtained in this scenario impact the physician or organization?

Resource

Klaver, J. C. 2017. Consent to Treatment. Chapter 8 in *Fundamentals of Law for Health Informatics and Information Management,* 3rd ed. M. S. Brodnik, L. A. Rinehart-Thompson, and R. B. Reynolds, eds. Chicago: AHIMA.

5.26 Labor and employment laws

Competency V.1

Assess Pine Valley Hospital's compliance with the following laws based on these scenarios.

1. **Equal Pay Act of 1963**
    Gertrude and Harry are both new coders at PVH. They have been hired at the entry level Coder 1 position; the position requires an associate degree, which they both recently earned. However, neither of them have previous HIM or coding experience. Gertrude will be working the first shift (day, 7 a.m. to 3 p.m.), while Harry works second shift (evening, 3 p.m. to 11 p.m.). Harry has achieved his CCS credential, but Gertrude has not. The rate of pay for Gertrude is $14.21 per hour; Harry will be making $14.71. Is the pay difference a violation of Equal Pay Act of 1963? Defend your response.

2. **Age Discrimination in Employment Act of 1967**
    Selena is the HIM director at a 200-bed hospital. She has had exemplary performance evaluations each of her 35 years (15 of which have been as director of HIM) and is a well-respected leader within the organization. Recent financial difficulties within the hospital have administration looking to cut costs. They have decided to dismiss Selena and hire a new director at a reduced salary and fringe benefits. In your opinion, does this violate the Age Discrimination Act? Again, defend your answer.

Resource

LeBlanc, M. M. 2020. Human Resources Management. Chapter 21 in *Health Information Management: Concepts, Principles, and Practice*, 6th ed. P. Oachs and A. Watters, eds. Chicago: AHIMA.

5.27 Healthcare policies

Competency V.4

Gretchen Murphy, an HIM professional, has been asked to participate in a community panel discussion on national healthcare policies as they relate to access, cost, and quality. Her focus will be on cost of care. Gretchen wants to provide information on at least three federal regulations that have had an impact on the cost of healthcare. Select three federal regulations with such an impact and provide a brief synopsis of the key points as they each relate to healthcare cost.

Resource

Rinehart-Thompson, L. A. 2017. Patient Rights and Responsibilities. Chapter 14 in *Fundamentals of Law for Health Informatics and Information Management,* 3rd ed. M. S. Brodnik, L. A. Rinehart-Thompson, and R. B. Reynolds. Chicago: AHIMA.

5.28 Sentinel events

Competency V.2

A

Apply the Joint Commission's definition of sentinel event to determine if the following are sentinel events or not.

1. Baby boy Brown is discharged to the Carmichael family.

2. Mrs. Richards has extensive cardiac damage from several myocardial infarctions, along with multiple comorbid conditions, and dies during cardiac bypass surgery.

3. Patient Smith leaves the emergency department against medical advice.

4. Patient Thomas leaves the emergency department against medical advice and two days later commits suicide.

5. Mr. Johnson comes to ER with abdominal pain two days after inguinal hernia surgery. A CT scan indicates there is a hemostat in the abdominal area of the surgery.

Resource

Joint Commission. 2019. Sentinel events. https://www.jointcommission.org/assets/1/18/Sentinel %20Event%20Policy.pdf.

5.29 Laboratory billing change

Competency V.5

In April, one of the most experienced outpatient coders at Forest View Hospital, Sandy, approaches you, her manager, to discuss a potential billing issue. Sandy noticed that since early March, the number of lab tests performed on outpatient referral accounts that she codes has increased significantly. As she began to pay more attention to this, she realized that that she wasn't seeing a basic metabolic panel (BMP) in the charges as often as she had been previously. What she was seeing reflected in the charges were all of the following instead: calcium, carbon dioxide, sodium, potassium, glucose, urea nitrogen, creatinine, and chloride.

You decide to begin an investigation by running a report for the use of the CPT code for a BMP (80047) from January through the current date of April 10th. The results indicate that prior to March 7th, BMP was coded 627 times, but from March 7th to April 10th, the number dropped dramatically, to just 75, with most of them in early March and fewer into April. Next, you ran a report to determine the number of billed accounts that included all eight tests under investigation. These results showed that prior to March 7th, there were no accounts that had all eight tests billed, but after that date, 237 accounts were billed with all eight tests.

You decide that you need to meet with the director of the lab in order to get to the bottom of this change. This will be your first meeting with Josie, the lab director, who was just hired at the end of February.

1. Provide an interpretation of the report results that are provided and what problem they signify.

2. Recommend a strategy to correct the problem detected.

Reference

Hunt, T. J. and K. Kirk. 2020. Clinical Documentation Improvement and Coding Compliance. Chapter 9 in *Health Information Management: Concepts, Principles, and Practice*, 6th ed. P. Oachs and A. Watters, eds. Chicago: AHIMA.

5.30 ICD-10-CM notes

Competency V.5

Prior to October 1, 2017, there was an ICD-10-CM coding note at J44.0 COPD with acute lower respiratory infection that stated "Use additional code to identify infection." This dictated the sequencing of the COPD with pneumonia, as any patient admitted with both conditions POA (present on admission) must be sequenced with the pneumonia as the secondary diagnosis. On October 1, 2017, that note was changed to read "Code also to identify infection." Since that time, Alice, the previous coding supervisor, directed her coding staff to assign pneumonia as the principal diagnosis on all those accounts when both COPD and pneumonia were POA.

Shortly after your hiring as Alice's replacement, one of the coders approaches you with concerns about this directive. Assess the problems this directive has created and then provide a better interpretation of the note change for your coding staff.

Reference

Hunt, T. J. and K. Kirk. 2020. Clinical Documentation Improvement and Coding Compliance. Chapter 9 in *Health Information Management: Concepts, Principles, and Practice*, 6th ed. P. Oachs and A. Watters, eds. Chicago: AHIMA.

5.31 Attempted medical identity theft

Competency V.5

Last week, a case of attempted external medical identity theft was uncovered in the physician's practice where you are the office manager. You had been speaking with a patient, and repeated their full name back to them for clarification as you entered it in the EHR, when one of the medical assistants walked by. He motioned to speak with you in private and communicated that the patient was not who he said he was. You returned to the patient requesting additional verification of identity like a credit card or driver's license, but the patient got flustered and left the office.

Later that afternoon, you shared the encounter with the physician, who wanted to know what processes were in place to prevent that from happening again. Unfortunately, there was nothing currently in place, but you assure him that you will look into the options, establish some policies and procedures, and educate the staff.

Propose at least five options, both electronic and paper-based, that can be put into place to mitigate the likelihood that external medical identity theft would go unnoticed.

Reference

Olenik, K. and R. B. Reynolds. 2017. Security Threats and Controls. Chapter 13 in *Fundamentals of Law for Health Informatics and Information Management*, 3rd ed. M. S. Brodnik, L. A. Rinehart-Thompson, and R. B. Reynolds, eds. Chicago: AHIMA.

5.32 Claim review—blockchain

Competency V.5

You have begun work for a health insurer as an emergency department claims reviewer. Your focus is physician level 5 emergency department visits billed with CPT code 99285. Over the course of your training, you recognize that one physician has a much higher percentage of level 5 visits than the other doctors. You take this information to your supervisor, who runs a report that substantiates your findings, with that physician having more than three times as many level 5 visits as any other physician. Further investigation shows that the documentation for these visits is eerily similar, with whole sections that are identical, signaling that the documentation may be fraudulent.

Your supervisor initiates a full review of the medical records for all the billed level 5 accounts from that physician, which turns out to be very time consuming. However, the time is well spent, as you are able to identify that the physician has been going back into the dictation and adding information to fraudulently boost the level.

You wonder if there is a more efficient way to be proactive in identifying and tracking this type of fraud. You recall reading about blockchain technology in a recent *Journal of AHIMA* article and think that might be a useful tool.

Propose to your supervisor the benefits of blockchain technology and ways this technology can be leveraged to prevent this type of fraud in the future. Additionally, create a staff-training memo that outlines this technology to ensure everyone is familiar with this technology.

References

Parks, L. 2019. Is Blockchain Technology in Your Revenue Cycle Future? https://journal.ahima.org /2019/02/12/is-blockchain-technology-in-your-revenue-cycle-future/

Viola, A. 2018. Blockchain's Role in Health IT. *Journal of AHIMA* 89(9): 34–35, 54.

5.33 Modifier 25 denials

Competency V.5

As the patient accounting and HIM director at a small, critical access hospital, you review the denials and account issues that arise for both the facility and the providers for whom you bill. Two years ago, you were looking at emergency department (ED) provider claims that had procedures performed. In every case, an E&M level code had been assigned in addition to the procedure, and all E&Ms had been assigned modifier 25, which enabled them to bypass the edit stating that without the modifier, the E&M level would not be paid. As you pulled the records of these accounts, you realize that not all of them met the criteria to have the modifier 25 added. Further investigation showed that staff in patient accounting had added the modifiers once the billing scrubber kicked them back. You told them that this was inappropriate and could be construed as fraud and then explained that modifier 25 indicted that the E&M was unrelated to the procedure. That would mean that some other condition would have to be addressed during the visit, which was not always the case. A good example was the patients who come for laceration repairs without any further workup. These should only generate the procedure code, no E&M level.

After educating the staff and making corrections to what had been billed incorrectly, you reviewed claims for a month to ensure that the staff were complying with the new directions. All appeared well.

Last week, you looked at several ED provider claims on an unrelated issue but discovered this same issue had reappeared as well. Confused by this, you speak to the billers and discover that a new biller, hired six months ago, had added the modifier 25. He indicates that this was the procedure at his previous place of employment and, without any direction otherwise, he had carried that process over to this position.

Recommend strategies that could be implemented to ensure that this error does not continue to happen.

Reference

Casto, A. B. 2018. *Principles of Healthcare Reimbursement,* 6th ed. Chicago: AHIMA.

Chapter 6

Domain VI: Organizational Management and Leadership

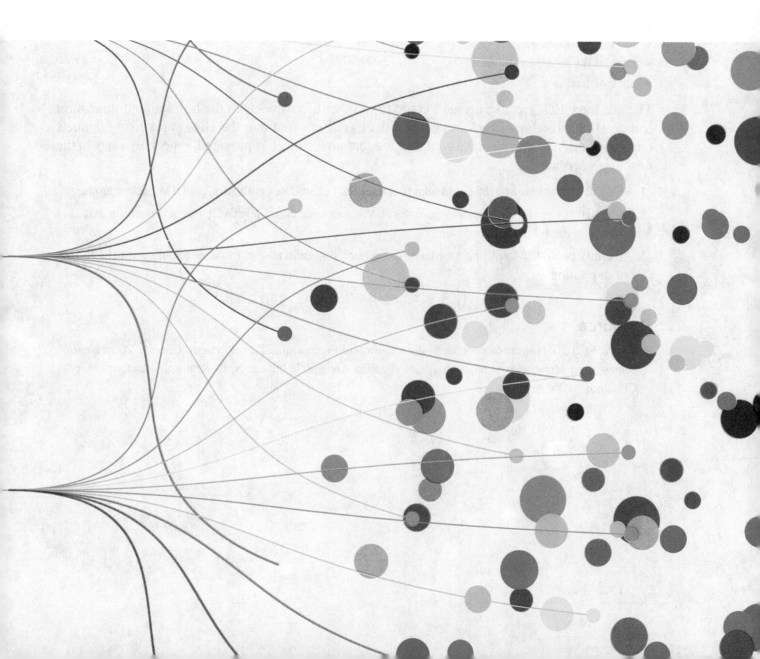

6.0 Release of information for employee training and development

A

Competency VI.3

Competency VI.5

Competency VI.9

Martha, the HIM director for Richmond Medical Center, has lost her third release of information (ROI) technician in the past year. It seems as though shortly after the new hires pass the probationary period, they quit. Exit interviews have provided the following information:

- Job is too stressful (unfamiliar with HIPAA regulations, backlog high)
- Job is too much for one person
- Job is too confusing
- Lack of departmental training
- Lack of feedback

The last three ROI technicians have come from other departments in the hospital, but none have had an HIM educational background. Martha has discovered that the HIM supervisor conducts one day of orientation and one day of training, but no feedback is provided, especially early in the new hire's service.

1. Decide what steps Martha could take to attract ROI candidates with stronger HIM backgrounds.
2. Identify at least four key areas where the HIM supervisor could positively impact retention and select methods for that improvement.
3. Identify two other steps that Martha or the supervisor could take to improve retention for the ROI tech position.

Resource

Prater, V. S. 2020. Human Resources Management and Professional Development. Chapter 20 in *Health Information Management Technology: An Applied Approach*, 6th ed. N. B. Sayles and L. Gordon, eds. Chicago: AHIMA.

6.1 Committee consensus

Competency VI.1

Norwood Health Services just acquired two new hospitals as part of its system, which already had two acute care facilities. You are the HIM director of one of new hospitals and serve on the corporate HIM committee along with the other three HIM directors. The original two acute care facilities have been dual-coding outpatient records with both ICD-10-CM and PCS codes, while your facility and the other recently acquired hospital have not. It is imperative to arrive at a consensus at today's meeting as to whether dual coding should be done at all four facilities, as the corporate HIM director wants to standardize corporate strategy. One of the sticking points in the decision-making process has been report writing. One director is adamant that using the ICD-10-PCS codes will be the only way to capture the data for certain reports. Another director wants the benefit of cross-trained staff.

1. Provide at least three arguments you can present to influence those directors to join your position against transitioning all outpatient coders on ICD-10-PCS.

2. Propose a plan of action that might achieve a consensus.

Resources

HCPro. 2013. Outpatient coding and ICD-10-PCS. *HIM-HIPAA Insider*. http://www.hcpro.com /HIM-298135-865/Outpatient-coding-and-ICD10PCS.html.

York, M. 2015. To code or not to code-PCS codes on outpatient claims. *Libman Education* blog. http:// www.libmaneducation.com/to-code-or-not-to-code-pcs-codes-on-outpatient-claims/.

6.2 Transcription performance improvement

Competency VI.4

The head surgical nurse has expressed to you, an HIM director, her concerns regarding the lack of H&Ps on patients' charts, which causes surgical delays. Since a patient is not permitted to go to surgery without an H&P on record, this is causing serious issues, including daily backlogs or cancellations. Patients are becoming angry and surgeons want something done to eliminate this issue.

1. Plan a data collection to assess the situation, selecting the relevant data elements to be included.

2. Identify any other information that may be pertinent to the evaluation of the data collection from the transcription standpoint.

3. Assume that the data collected identifies one particular physician who has this issue repeatedly. His surgeries are scheduled beginning at 6:00 a.m. and he routinely dictates the H&Ps starting at 5:50 a.m. What strategies can be developed to reduce the delays?

Resource

Shaw P. L. and D. Carter. 2019. *Quality and Performance Improvement in Healthcare: A Tool for Programmed Learning*, 7th ed. Chicago: AHIMA.

6.3 Ethical situation

Competency VI.7

Since May, you have been working with a recruiter to obtain a new position in HIM. Your experience includes over ten years in inpatient and outpatient coding, you are an AHIMA-approved ICD-10 trainer, and you have worked with your state association on coding projects over the past two years. Nothing the recruiter has presented to you has been a good fit, but in late September, the recruiter calls with positions open for coding auditor. You have never done that type of work before, but are confident you could learn, and the recruiter gets you a phone interview. During the conversation, the HIM manager for the organization says that she sees you have been an auditor since May. You immediately recognize that the HIM manager has the wrong impression of your experience.

Determine the appropriate course of action in response to the interviewer's statement. Provide justification based on the AHIMA Code of Ethics.

Resource

AHIMA. 2019. AHIMA Code of Ethics. http://bok.ahima.org/doc?oid=105098#.XR-TMOtKi71.

A

B

6.4 Ethics breach

Competency VI.7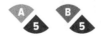

Your regional HIM association has enlisted a speaker on privacy and security based on the presentation experience listed on her resume. Immediately after the presentation, several members approach you to say they are certain that today's presentation was exactly the same one that they had attended at the state association meeting two years ago given by a different speaker. Assess the implications for this individual if she breached ethical standards by passing off someone else's work as her own.

Resources

AHIMA. 2019a. AHIMA Code of Ethics. http://bok.ahima.org/doc?oid=105098#.XR-TMOtKi71.

AHIMA. 2019b. Policy and Procedure for Disciplinary Review and Appeal. http://www.ahima.org
/downloads/AHIMA_%20RevisedDISCIPLINARYREVIEWAPPEALS1-9-19.pdf.

6.5 Ethical dilemma

Competency VI.7

As HIM director of Pine Valley Community Hospital, a critical access hospital, you are concerned about a recent decision made by your CEO. He has decided that all patients will be issued an Advanced Beneficiary Notice for outpatient laboratory and radiology services. His rationale is that by doing this, the hospital will be able to collect on all the tests performed that do not meet medical necessity. You know that is an unacceptable practice.

1. Defend your position.
2. Support your stance through the Code of Ethics.
3. Anticipate the consequences of continuing with the CEO's decision.

Resources

AHIMA. 2019. AHIMA Code of Ethics. http://bok.ahima.org/doc?oid=105098#.XR-TMOtKi71.

Centers for Medicare and Medicaid Services. 2018. Medicare Advance Beneficiary Notices. https://www.cms.gov/Outreach-and-Education/Medicare-Learning-Network-MLN/MLNProducts /downloads/abn_booklet_icn006266.pdf.

Centers for Medicare and Medicaid Services. 2019. Time Limits and Penalties for Physicians and Suppliers in Making Refunds. Medicare Claims Processing Manual. https://www.cms.gov/Medicare /Medicare-General-Information/BNI/Downloads/ABN-CMS-Manual-Instructions.pdf.

6.6 Ethical decision-making

Competency VI.7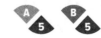

An inpatient coder has come to you, the director of HIM, with concerns that she has been instructed by the coding supervisor to code all bedside debridements as excisional. When you discuss this with the coding supervisor, she explains that surgical trays are ordered for the bedside and that physicians have been ignoring the queries requesting clarification. Instead, they orally state that the debridements are always excisional. Therefore, she issued the directive to the staff.

1. Use the ethical decision-making process to determine if this is an unethical situation and, if so, what principle of the AHIMA Code of Ethics or AHIMA's Standards of Ethical Coding it violates.

2. If it is a violation, give your opinion of what the implications might be to the coder, coding supervisor, yourself, and the organization.

Resources

AHIMA. 2019. AHIMA Code of Ethics. http://bok.ahima.org/doc?oid=105098#.XR-TMOtKi71.

AHIMA. 2016. AHIMA Standards of Ethical Coding. http://bok.ahima.org/CodingStandards# .XFn1KFVKi70.

Hamilton, M. 2020. Ethical Issues in Health Information Management. Chapter 21 in *Health Information Management Technology: An Applied Approach*, 6th ed. N. B. Sayles and L. Gordon, eds. Chicago: AHIMA.

Swirsky, E. 2020. Ethical Issues in Health Information Management. Chapter X in *Health Information Management: Concepts, Principles, and Practice*, 6th ed. P. Oachs and A. Watters, eds. Chicago: AHIMA.

6.7 Preparing for an HIM job interview

Competency VI.3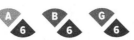

Imagine you are preparing for your first job interview in an HIM department. You are trying to prepare answers to likely interview questions. You are comfortable discussing everything on your resume, including your education and previous non–HIM related work experience. You have thought about what strengths and weaknesses you have and recalled a couple experiences that can illustrate your work ethic. You even role-play with a friend to reduce your anxiety, except you are thrown a curve when the first thing she says to you is "tell me a little about yourself."

1. Compose an appropriate response to this question.

2. Hypothesize why an HIM director might ask such a question.

Resources

LeBlanc, M. M. 2020. Human Resources Management. Chapter 22 in *Health Information Management: Concepts, Principles, and Practice*, 6th ed. P. Oachs and A. Watters, eds. Chicago: AHIMA.

Prater, V. S. 2020. Human Resources Management and Professional Development. Chapter 20 in *Health Information Management Technology: An Applied Approach*, 6th ed. N. B. Sayles and L. Gordon, eds. Chicago: AHIMA.

6.8 HIM job interview

Competency VI.3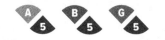

Evaluate the following interchange between an HIM director and prospective employee. Critique the questions asked by the HIM director and identify any that are inappropriate to ask during the interview process and explain why.

HIM director: Welcome, Ms. Martin. I'm Sheila Reynolds, HIM director. I see from your resume that you just completed the HIT program at Wentworth College. Tell me about your favorite class.

Ms. Martin: I really enjoyed the three coding classes that I took. I found them to be challenging but fun. Those classes had me utilizing my anatomy and physiology knowledge as well.

HIM director: Indeed. As I reviewed your resume, I noticed there is a 10-year time lapse between your last job and returning to college. Can you explain that? Were you taking time to start a family?

Ms. Martin: Yes; now that my children are older, I am more comfortable getting back into the work force.

HIM director: There are times throughout the year when our staff must put in overtime. Do you have after school childcare lined up?

Ms. Martin: There is an afterschool program at the school itself that they will attend. I think it will work out well.

HIM director: Can you tell me what your greatest strength is?

Ms. Martin: I would say that I am a very conscientious person. I like to do a good job at whatever I do and work hard to learn when I have made a mistake.

HIM director: Then what would be your greatest weakness?

Ms. Martin: I would have to say that I am impatient; however, the advantage to that is that I like to get things done quickly.

HIM director: How are you with multi-tasking?

Ms. Martin: I worked part-time while going to school and raising my kids. I had to multi-task every day in order to keep everyone on schedule. I never was late for work or turned in a late assignment.

HIM director: Didn't your husband help out?

Ms. Martin: We are divorced.

HIM director: Okay, well, tell me how you would handle a physician who comes into the department yelling about having to redictate several operative reports.

Ms. Martin: First, I would ask him to step into an office for a private discussion. Then I would listen to his complaints. I would tell him that I would investigate his concerns about the transcription system and explain that in the meantime, we really will have to ask him to dictate the reports again.

HIM director: Thank you, Ms. Martin. I have a few more interviews and will be in touch by the end of the week with my decision.

Ms. Martin: Thank you, Ms. Reynolds. I appreciate the opportunity to interview for the coding position and look forward to hearing from you soon. Goodbye.

Resources

LeBlanc, M. M. 2020. Human Resources Management. Chapter 22 in *Health Information Management: Concepts, Principles, and Practice*, 6th ed. P. Oachs and A. Watters, eds. Chicago: AHIMA.

Prater, V. S. 2020. Human Resources Management and Professional Development. Chapter 20 in *Health Information Management Technology: An Applied Approach*, 6th ed. N. B. Sayles and L. Gordon, eds. Chicago: AHIMA.

6.9 Calculating release of information staffing levels

Competency VI.3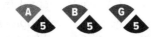

Determine the number of full-time release of information (ROI) staff that is needed for an HIM department based on the following information. Use a 7.5-hour work day for your calculation. On average, ROI clerks process the following:

Open and log all the mail (average of 16 pieces of mail per day)

Of those 5 per day are attorney requests—35 minutes to complete and log

5 per week are subpoenas—2.5 hours to complete and log

9 per day are insurance requests—45 minutes to complete and log

1 miscellaneous request per day—30 minutes to complete and log

20 walk-in requests per day—10 minutes to complete and log requests

Resource

Horton, L. A. 2017. *Calculating and Reporting Healthcare Statistics, Revised Reprint,* 5th ed. Chicago: AHIMA.

6.10 Coder education

Competency VI.3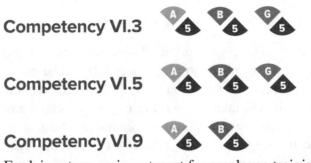

Competency VI.5

Competency VI.9

Explain return on investment for employee training and development.

Budget planning is underway in your organization, and as HIM director, you are preparing the budgets for your department. A memo accompanied the annual worksheets for capital and operational budgets stating that all educational expenses were being cut this year. In past years, you have budgeted $2,500 for coding education, which included sending two coders to your state association's annual meeting for the coding day presentations ($250 for both including travel), purchase of five AHIMA coding webinars ($750 total, $150 each), resource books ($250) and registration and travel for one person to the annual AHIMA conference ($1,250). Draft a memo to your boss, Mary Winters, CFO, and defend the necessity of keeping coding education in your budget.

Resources

Gordon, L. 2020. Management. Chapter 17 in *Health Information Management Technology: An Applied Approach*, 6th ed. N. B. Sayles and L. Gordon, eds. Chicago: AHIMA.

Patena, K. 2020. Employee Training and Development. Chapter 23 in *Health Information Management: Concepts, Principles, and Practice*, 6th ed. P. Oachs and A. Watters, eds. Chicago: AHIMA.

Prater, V. S. 2020. Human Resources Management and Professional Development. *Health Information Management Technology: An Applied Approach*, 6th ed. N. B. Sayles and L. Gordon, eds. Chicago: AHIMA.

Revoir, R. 2020. Financial Management. Chapter 25 in *Health Information Management: Concepts, Principles, and Practice*, 6th ed. P. Oachs and A. Watters, eds. Chicago: AHIMA.

6.11 New service impact on coding staff levels

Competency VI.3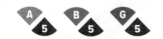

In July, a new endoscopy suite will be opened in your organization. Projections are that 60 endoscopies will be performed per day. At the same time, an electrophysiology lab will be opening, with anticipation of 5 procedures being done there per day. You have done some preliminary work sampling to determine how much time it will take to code these types of cases and arrived at 5 minutes per endoscopy and 15 minutes per EP procedure. Calculate the number of full-time equivalents (FTEs) that you will need to hire to cover the additional workload. Base your calculations on a 7.5-hour workday.

Resource

Horton, L. A. 2017. *Calculating and Reporting Healthcare Statistics,* 5th ed., revised reprint. Chicago: AHIMA.

6.12 New HIM roles

Competency VI.1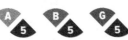

As a student, you recognize that the HIM profession is in a perpetual state of growth, with new opportunities on the horizon, and you are trying to decide what HIM niche is the right fit for you. Use the AHIMA career map to explore one of those emerging roles in HIM.

1. Judge what additional skills or education you would need to qualify for the new role.

2. Next, go to the AHIMA website and find information on the HIM Reimagined strategy. Assess how that emerging HIM role and skills it will require correlate with HIM Reimagined.

Resources

American Health Information Management Association. 2019. Health Information Careers. https:// my.ahima.org/careermap.

American Health Information Management Association. 2017. HIM Reimagined. https://www.ahima .org/about/him-reimagined/himr?tabid=whitepaper.

6.13 HIM and the C-suite

Competency VI.1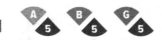

Laura is an RHIT who has been an HIM department director for the past five years, with much of her focus on release of information and revenue cycle. She wants to take her career to a new level using her skills related to HIPAA and coding/reimbursement. Laura knows that her organization is in the processing of creating some new C-suite positions and she would like to be in a position to be considered for them. Perform research on the healthcare C-suite positions that are available and select two that best coincide with Laura's skill set. Determine if Laura has the necessary AHIMA credential(s) that would correlate with the positions.

Resources

AHIMA. n.d.a. Certification. Accessed July 19, 2019. https://www.ahima.org/certification.

AHIMA. n.d.b. Health Information Careers. Accessed July 19, 2019. https://my.ahima.org/careermap.

Gordon, L. L. 2020. Leadership. Chapter 19 in *Health Information Management Technology: An Applied Approach*, 6th ed. N. B. Sayles and L. Gordon, eds. Chicago: AHIMA.

Sayles, N. B. 2020. Health Information Management Profession. Chapter 1 in *Health Information Management Technology: An Applied Approach*, 6th ed. N. B. Sayles and L. Gordon, eds. Chicago: AHIMA.

6.14 Cultural awareness self-assessment

Competency VI.6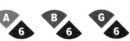

Michael is an HIM director at a local hospital in West Virginia. Michael recently ran reports on patient admissions by ethnicity and discovered that over the past three years, the Hispanic population has increased from 3 percent to 18 percent. When looking at patient satisfaction scores from that population, he noticed that the scores are much lower than normal.

1. Theorize what could be causing the low patient satisfaction scores from a cultural diversity standpoint.

2. Propose at least four measures the facility could implement that would foster cultural diversity.

3. Elaborate on at least three reasons why embracing cultural diversity would benefit the organization.

Resources

Hamilton, M. 2020. Ethical Issues in Health Information Management. Chapter 21 in *Health Information Management Technology: An Applied Approach*, 6th ed. N. B. Sayles and L. Gordon, eds. Chicago: AHIMA.

Swirsky, E. 2020. Ethical Issues in Health Information Management. Chapter 27 in *Health Information Management: Concepts, Principles, and Practice*, 6th ed. P. Oachs and A. Watters, eds. Chicago: AHIMA.

6.15 Americans with Disabilities Act and HIM

Competency VI.6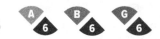

Margie is part of the human resources department at Oak Ridge Memorial Hospital and is currently reviewing applications for the open outpatient coding position. She has several candidates that meet all the qualifications and one final application for review. That individual has the most experience, 15 years as an outpatient coder at another facility, but has been out of work for two years. Margie calls her to set up an interview and, in the process, finds out that she is blind. There was an accident two years that took her eyesight completely. Once Margie hears that, she cancels the interview.

1. Is Margie's action appropriate or inappropriate based on the Americans with Disabilities Act (ADA)?

2. Are Margie's actions acceptable under the ADA if the applicant had reduced visibility rather than total blindness?

Resources

Hamilton, M. 2020. Ethical Issues in Health Information Management. Chapter 21 in *Health Information Management Technology: An Applied Approach*, 6th ed. N. B. Sayles and L. Gordon, eds. Chicago: AHIMA.

LeBlanc, M. 2020. Human Resources Management. Chapter 22 in *Health Information Management: Concepts, Principles, and Practice*, 6th ed. P. Oachs and A. Watters, eds. Chicago: AHIMA.

Patena, K. 2020. Employee Training and Development. Chapter 23 in *Health Information Management: Concepts, Principles, and Practice*, 6th ed. P. Oachs and A. Watters, eds. Chicago: AHIMA.

Prater, V. S. 2020. Human Resources Management and Professional Development. Chapter 20 in *Health Information Management Technology: An Applied Approach*, 6th ed. N. B. Sayles and L. Gordon, eds. Chicago: AHIMA.

Reynolds, R. B. and M. S. Brodnik. 2017. Workplace Law. Chapter 20 in *Fundamentals of Law for Health Informatics and Information Management,* 3rd ed. M. S. Brodnik, L. A. Rinehart-Thompson, and R. B. Reynolds, eds. Chicago: AHIMA.

6.16 HIM department diversity

Competency VI.6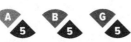

A 60-year-old woman has just been hired as the HIM director at an organization where a majority of her staff is in their early 20s, with many of them being recent graduates. Assess the cultural diversity that you would expect to be evident in the department and the potential challenges that the director might face.

Resources

Dimick, C. 2007. HIM manager, non-HIM staff: managing staff with expertise beyond HIM. *Journal of AHIMA* 78(9).

Patena, K. 2020. Employee Training and Development. Chapter 23 in *Health Information Management: Concepts, Principles, and Practice*, 6th ed. P. Oachs and A. Watters, eds. Chicago: AHIMA.

Swirsky, E. 2020. Ethical Issues in Health Information Management. Chapter 27 in *Health Information Management: Concepts, Principles, and Practice*, 6th ed. P. Oachs and A. Watters, eds. Chicago: AHIMA.

6.17 Art of negotiating

Competency VI.1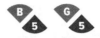

You are training an assistant to participate in organizational performance improvement committees. After observing the interaction at a recent meeting, the assistant states that the committee seems divided in two on how best to proceed and both sides are entrenched in their positions. He is unsure how to proceed to get the committee back on track. Recommend at least four strategies for negotiation that the assistant can employ.

Resources

Dimick, C. 2007. HIM manager, non-HIM staff: managing staff with expertise beyond HIM. *Journal of AHIMA* 78(9).

Patena, K. 2020. Employee Training and Development. Chapter 23 in *Health Information Management: Concepts, Principles, and Practice*, 6th ed. P. Oachs and A. Watters, eds. Chicago: AHIMA.

Swenson, D. X. 2020. Managing and Leading During Organization Change. Chapter 21 in *Health Information Management: Concepts, Principles, and Practice*, 6th ed. P. Oachs and A. Watters, eds. Chicago: AHIMA.

6.18 Salary negotiation

Competency VI.1

For the past three weeks you have been in the application and interview process for an HIM director position. You currently work as an assistant director at another area hospital and have 15 years of HIM experience. Today, you were offered the job with a salary that is comparable to what you make now. The organization is roughly the same size as the one where you are currently employed. You think that you should make more for the upper level position. Develop a strategy to address your salary concern and then formulate your response to the offer.

Resources

Dimick, C. 2007. HIM manager, non-HIM staff: Managing staff with expertise beyond HIM. *Journal of AHIMA* 78(9).

Kaplan-Quinn, G. 2003. New job? More money? Negotiating pays off. *Journal of AHIMA* 74(6):46.

LeBlanc, M. M. 2020. Human Resources Management. Chapter 22 in *Health Information Management: Concepts, Principles, and Practice*, 6th ed. P. Oachs and A. Watters, eds. Chicago: AHIMA.

B

G

6.19 Identify types of budget variances

Competency VI.5

Identify the following types of budget variances by indicating if they are temporary or permanent and favorable or unfavorable.

1. $7,500.00 for outsourced coding services to address backlog after a coder took an unexpected leave for six weeks

2. $12,500.00 as a result of assistant director laid off in November

3. $500 for new computer needed to replace one that quit and was not repairable

4. $4,000.00 1st quarter record destruction postponed a quarter due to staffing issues

Resources

Gordon, L. 2020. Management. Chapter 17 in *Health Information Management Technology: An Applied Approach*, 6th ed. N. B. Sayles and L. Gordon, eds. Chicago: AHIMA.

Revoir, R. 2020. Financial Management. Chapter 25 in *Health Information Management: Concepts, Principles, and Practice*, 6th ed. P. Oachs and A. Watters, eds. Chicago: AHIMA.

6.20 Depreciation

Competency VI.5

HIM director Kimberly Pierce is hoping to budget for new office furniture for her staff. She has done some preliminary calculations to determine how much she will need and has determined that she needs to budget $10,000. Her chief financial officer has asked her to calculate the straight line depreciation for the office furniture, assuming there will be a residual value of $2,000. He agrees the useful life of the furniture is 10 years.

Resources

Revoir, R. 2020. Financial Management. Chapter 25 in *Health Information Management: Concepts, Principles, and Practice*, 6th ed. P. Oachs and A. Watters, eds. Chicago: AHIMA.

White. S. 2018. Understanding Financial Statements. Chapter 2 in *Principles of Finance for Health Information and Informatics Professionals*, 2nd ed. Chicago, AHIMA.

6.21 Hospital merger

Competency VI.2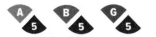

Two local hospitals that are struggling financially have decided to merge. Consolidation of services, including HIM, will be taking place. Examine the two HIM department structures in place now and offer an opinion about how they could be restructured. Be sure to support your position.

Hospital 1	**Hospital 2**
Director	Director
Department supervisor	Transcription supervisor
Transcription supervisor	4 coders
8 coders	5 transcriptionists
12 transcriptionists	2 assemblers/analysts
6 assemblers/analysts	1 ROI clerk
2 ROI clerks	1 full-time and 1 part-time scanner tech
3 scanner techs	1 incomplete records
2 incomplete records	4 file clerks
4 file clerks	1 cancer registrar
1 cancer registrar	

Resources

AHIMA. 2012. Identifying Issues in Facility and Provider Mergers and Acquisitions. *Journal of AHIMA* 83(2): 50–53.

Gordon, L. 2020. Management. Chapter 17 in *Health Information Management Technology: An Applied Approach*, 6th ed. N. B. Sayles and L. Gordon, eds. Chicago: AHIMA.

LeBlanc, M. M. 2020. Human Resources Management. Chapter 22 in *Health Information Management: Concepts, Principles, and Practice*, 6th ed. P. Oachs and A. Watters, eds. Chicago: AHIMA.

Prater, V. S. 2020. Human Resources Management and Professional Development. Chapter 20 in *Health Information Management Technology: An Applied Approach*, 6th ed. N. B. Sayles and L. Gordon, eds. Chicago: AHIMA.

Swenson, D. 2020. Managing and Leading During Organization Changes. Chapter 21 in *Health Information Management: Concepts, Principles, and Practice*, 6th ed. P. Oachs and A. Watters, eds. Chicago: AHIMA.

6.22 Benchmarking performance

Competency VI.3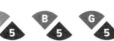

You have six scanner techs. Three work first shift (D), three work second shift (A), and each is assigned to a specific scanner, noted below. A scanning backlog is growing over the past week, so you have decided to evaluate their productivity. They each recorded their daily productivity over the past two weeks. Since they do not have other department responsibilities, all their time is spent on scanning. One staff member, Teresa, worked a half day on one of the days, and one person, John, had a personal day; otherwise, the techs all worked their full 8-hour shift daily for the two-week period under study.

Scanner ID	Employee	Total # of scanned records
Scanner 1(D)	John	112,892
Scanner 2(D)	Teresa	160,588
Scanner 3(D)	Larry	193,248
Scanner 1(A)	Mary	138,800
Scanner 2(A)	Jenny	182,160
Scanner 3(A)	Tom	184,960

1. Calculate each tech's hourly productivity as well as an overall group productivity.

2. Determine if the individuals and group are meeting the benchmark of 1,200 to 2,400 scanned images per hour.

3. What conclusions can you draw from this study?

4. Recommend a new productivity standard based on the information gathered above in order to reduce the backlog.

5. If your scanning backlog has been about 1,000 pages per day, under the new productivity standard, how long will it take to erase the backlog?

6. Do you have enough staff to handle the current workload if there is no backlog?

Resources

Dunn, R. 2007. Benchmarking imaging: Making every image count in scanning programs. *Journal of AHIMA* 78(6):42–46.

LeBlanc, M. M. 2020. Human Resources Management. Chapter 22 in *Health Information Management: Concepts, Principles, and Practice*, 6th ed. P. Oachs and A. Watters, eds. Chicago: AHIMA.

Prater, V. S. 2020. Human Resources Management and Professional Development. Chapter 20 in *Health Information Management Technology: An Applied Approach*, 6th ed. N. B. Sayles and L. Gordon, eds. Chicago: AHIMA.

Swenson, D. 2020. Managing and Leading During Organization Changes. Chapter 21 in *Health Information Management: Concepts, Principles, and Practice*, 6th ed. P. Oachs and A. Watters, eds. Chicago: AHIMA.

6.23 Vendor selection

Competency VI.1

Your organization is going to implement a new EHR. During the vendor selection process, five vendors are recognized as potential suppliers. Three of the vendors are well-known companies; the other two are smaller companies.

1. Identify at least five criteria that you would expect to be used in the decision-making process.

2. Explain why cost should not be the determining factor when choosing an EHR vendor.

Resource

Amatayakul, M. K. 2017. *Heath IT and EHRs Principles and Practice*, 6th ed. Chicago: AHIMA.

6.24 Project management life cycle

Competency VI.1

Susan volunteers for her state HIM association and heads the committee that is in charge of enlisting speakers on coding topics for the annual meeting. Her committee has lined up four speakers to deliver presentations. Three days before the event, the president of the state association calls Susan to say that one of the speakers has not submitted his presentation so handouts can be made. Susan emails the speaker and gets an out-of-office email in return stating the speaker is on vacation for the next week and will respond upon his return. Susan telephones the speaker to verify his participation at the meeting, but learns the speaker is out of the country and will not return in time to present. He states he emailed about his unavailability six weeks ago. Susan is now in a panic since they are short one speaker for the day.

1. Identify the project management process that Susan failed to incorporate for this event.

2. As a member of the committee, take part in a brainstorming session to submit at least three options for consideration to fill the now empty speaker slot.

Resources

Gordon, L. 2020. Management. Chapter 17 in *Health Information Management Technology: An Applied Approach*, 6th ed. N. B. Sayles and L. Gordon, eds. Chicago: AHIMA.

Olson, B. 2020. Project Management. Chapter 26 in *Health Information Management: Concepts, Principles, and Practice*, 6th ed. P. Oachs and A. Watters. Chicago: AHIMA.

A

6.25 Emergency plan training

Competency VI.9

The HIM director has asked you to train the HIM staff on departmental responsibilities when a Code Adam (missing child) is announced. Without getting into specifics, devise a plan that would appeal to each type of sensory learner (visual, auditory, and kinesthetic).

Resources

Patena, K. 2020. Employee Training and Development. Chapter 23 in *Health Information Management: Concepts, Principles, and Practice*, 6th ed. P. Oachs and A. Watters, eds. Chicago: AHIMA.

Prater, V. S. 2020. Human Resources Management and Professional Development. Chapter 20 in *Health Information Management Technology: An Applied Approach*, 6th ed. N. B. Sayles and L. Gordon, eds. Chicago: AHIMA.

6.26 Team facilitator

Competency VI.1

You have been asked to be a team facilitator for a process improvement (PI) project for the HIM department. This is the first time for you to participate at this level as a team member. You understand PI processes and the tools used to achieve goals and are a good communicator. However, you are concerned that you may not have the interpersonal skills necessary to be a good facilitator.

1. Describe the facilitator's role in the team and determine how interpersonal skills are used.

2. Share your opinion on how important interpersonal skills would be in a facilitator role and why.

Resource

Shaw, P. L. and D. Carter. 2019. *Quality and Performance Improvement in Healthcare, A Tool for Programmed Learning,* 7th ed. Chicago: AHIMA.

6.27 Work redesign

Competency VI.1

Competency VI.2

Competency VI.10

As coding supervisor, you want to institute remote coding at your facility. With an EHR in place, you feel this would be an opportune time to develop this program. Your director has asked for a report on the work redesign needed in order for this transition to occur. Create a memo to director Margaret Smythe outlining the areas to be addressed and predict the level of difficulty that could be associated with each.

Resources

Coplan-Gould, W., K. Carolan, and B. Friedman. 2011. Re-engineering the coding workflow: Assessing today with an Eye toward tomorrow. *Journal of AHIMA* 82(7):20–24.

Hunt, T. J. and K. Kirk. 2020. Clinical Documentation Improvement and Coding Compliance. Chapter 9 in *Health Information Management: Concepts, Principles, and Practice*, 6th ed. P. Oachs and A. Watters, eds. Chicago: AHIMA.

Knight, B. and E. Lewis. 2004. *Three Steps to Remote Coding Success: The Sun Health Experience*. AHIMA Communities of Practice.

6.28 Mentor

Competency VI.1

As the coding supervisor at your organization, a file clerk who would like to become a coder has approached you. She has an associate degree in health information management, but she needs a mentor to help her reach her goal. Propose at least four steps that she can take to help her achieve her goal.

Resource

Patena, K. 2020. Employee Training and Development. Chapter 23 in *Health Information Management: Concepts, Principles, and Practice*, 6th ed. P. Oachs and A. Watters, eds. Chicago: AHIMA.

B

G

6.29 Coding productivity standards

Competency VI.3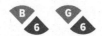

As the newly hired coding manager at your 300-bed acute-care facility, you are surprised that there are no coding productivity standards in place. Your organization outsources the same-day surgery accounts, but everything else is coded internally with the number of charts per coder varying greatly. Unfortunately, the discharged not final billed amount is climbing at an alarming rate. In an effort to reduce the DNFB, you determine that coding productivity standards must be implemented. You benchmark against three local hospitals to set the standards. Their standards per day are:

	Inpatient	ER	Same day surgery	Ancillaries
Hospital A	30	150	60	265
Hospital B	18	90	40	250
Hospital C	27	120	50	275

Theorize at least four reasons why there is such a discrepancy in the productivity standards among these facilities.

Resource

Oachs, P. 2020. Work Design and Process Improvement. Chapter 25 in *Health Information Management: Concepts, Principles, and Practice*, 6th ed. P. Oachs and A. Watters, eds. Chicago: AHIMA.

6.30 Workflow design

Competency VI.2

Study the workflow illustrated below, which shows the movement of discharged charts in the HIM department once they are collected from patient floors on night shift. Recommend changes to the workflow that would streamline the process.

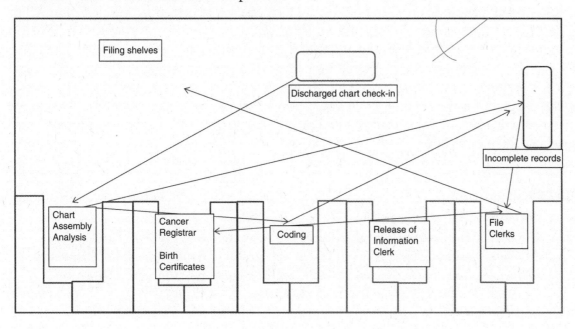

Resource

Oachs, P. 2020. Work Design and Process Improvement. Chapter 24 in *Health Information Management: Concepts, Principles, and Practice*, 6th ed. P. Oachs and A. Watters, eds. Chicago: AHIMA.

6.31 Swimlane diagram

Competency VI.2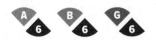

As the newly hired revenue cycle manager for Oak Ridge Hospital, you have been reviewing the revenue cycle process from start to finish. Issues are evident throughout the process. In the registration area, insurance information is not being verified, resulting in the patient accounting department having to request that registration contact the patient for correction prior to billing. The coding department finds issues with the patient admit status, especially for observation patients or outpatients that have an inpatient only procedure. Patient accounting is not only receiving denials for charges that are incorrectly entered for patients but prior to billing they have to contact the coding department for medical necessity edits which are found in the prebill scrubber. Create a swimlane diagram for the revenue cycle process covering the basic steps from registration to closing the patient account. Then, using a different colored arrow, show the issues in the process that have been identified above.

Resources

Handlon, L. 2020. Revenue Cycle Management. Chapter 8 in *Health Information Management: Concepts, Principles, and Practice*, 6th ed. P. Oachs and A. Watters, eds. Chicago: AHIMA.

Oachs, P. 2020. Work Design and Process Improvement. Chapter 24 in *Health Information Management: Concepts, Principles, and Practice*, 6th ed. P. Oachs and A. Watters, eds. Chicago: AHIMA.

6.32 Disciplinary action

Competency VI.3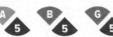

Assess the following situations and determine the disciplinary action that should be taken in each circumstance and justify your response.

1. One of your best inpatient coders was found to have violated HIPAA by looking at a physician's emergency department record. Investigation into that breach also found that he has accessed records of relatives and neighbors.

2. An audit of the file clerks has found that one clerk is making errors when filing loose sheets. They are not being incorporated into the correct chart. This same error was verbally addressed with the file clerk at her last performance evaluation two months ago.

3. On Saturday, your release of information clerk left the office open and unattended while she went to the restroom, which is against departmental policy. The nursing administrator on duty reported this to you as she had come to the office to request her recent lab results.

Resources

LeBlanc, M. M. 2020. Human Resources Management. Chapter 22 in *Health Information Management: Concepts, Principles, and Practice*, 6th ed. P. Oachs and A. Watters, eds. Chicago: AHIMA.

Prater, V. S. 2020. Human Resources Management and Professional Development. Chapter 20 in *Health Information Management Technology: An Applied Approach*, 6th ed. N. B. Sayles and L. Gordon, eds. Chicago: AHIMA.

A

B

G

6.33 Coder orientation

Competency VI.3

Competency VI.9

Laura is the coding supervisor at Oak Ridge Hospital. Her director informed her that administration has approved a new outpatient coder position, so the hiring process will begin soon. Laura has been directed to propose the topics that should be included in a department-specific orientation for the new coding staff member. Put yourself in her place and create that proposal. Also, choose one of the topics and suppose, it was not covered during the orientation process, what would or could happen?

Resources

Patena, K. 2020. Employee Training and Development. Chapter 23 in *Health Information Management: Concepts, Principles, and Practice*, 6th ed. P. Oachs and A. Watters, eds. Chicago: AHIMA.

Prater, V. S. 2020. Human Resources Management and Professional Development. Chapter 20 in *Health Information Management Technology: An Applied Approach*, 6th ed. N. B. Sayles and L. Gordon, eds. Chicago: AHIMA.

6.34 Request for information, request for proposal, and budget

Competency VI.1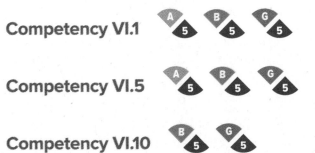

Competency VI.5

Competency VI.10

Your organization is considering outsourcing all of its coding services. Currently, coding staff use the 3M encoder and a computer-assisted coding program. The first step is to issue a request for information (RFI).

1. Evaluate the following results from your RFI and decide which three vendors to contact for a request for proposal (RFP).

	Turnaround Time		Are Coders Certified? AHIMA/ AAPC		Are Coders Familiar with 3M Encoder?		Are Coders Familiar with Computer Assisted Coding?		What Coding Services are Provided?				Payment?	
			Yes	No	Yes	No	Yes	No	Inpatient	Outpatient	Emergency	Ancillary	Per Chart	Per Hour
Vendor 1	48 hrs.		X		X		X		X	X	X	X	X	
Vendor 2	48 hrs.			X	X			X	X	X	X	X		X
Vendor 3	24 hrs.			X	X		X		X	X	X	X	X	
Vendor 4	72 hrs.		X		X		X		X	X	X	X		X
Vendor 5	48 hrs.		X		X		X		X	X	X	X		X

2. Now, determine eight items that should be included in the RFP that will be distributed.

3. Assume that you want to go with vendor 1 after the RFPs are evaluated. Now you must perform a cost-benefit analysis to see if it is feasible to entirely outsource. Their pricing structure is $5 per inpatient chart, $3 per outpatient chart, $1.75 for each ER, and $1 per ancillary account. Base your calculations on the average daily accounts for each patient type listed below:

Inpatient	70
Outpatient	75
Emergency Department	185
Ancillary	360

4. Now calculate your coding budget for next year. All full-time equivalent (FTE) staff will be getting a 2.5 percent raise; part-time (PT) staff will be getting 1 percent. In addition, you must also account for the fringe benefit costs associated with the coding staff, which are 32 percent of their salary. Calculations should be based on full-time employees working 40 hours per week with all part-time employees working half-time or 20 hours per week.

Coder	Current Rate	This Year's Salary	Raise	Next Year's Salary
Inpatient Coder 1 FTE	24.00 per hr.			
Inpatient Coder 2 FTE	22.50 per hr.			
Inpatient Coder 3 FTE	21.85 per hr.			
Outpatient Coder 1 FTE	19.75 per hr.			
Outpatient Coder 2 FTE	19.75 per hr.			
ER Coder 1 FTE	18.25 per hr.			
ER Coder 2 PT	18.25 per hr.			
Ancillary Coder 1 FTE	17.50 per hr.			
Ancillary Coder 2 PT	17.50 per hr.			

5. Is it cost effective to consider outsourcing coding based on these results?

6. What would the outcome be if you considered Vendor 5 at $30.00 per hour? (Use an eight-hour workday as your basis.)

Resources

Amatayakul, M. A. 2020. Health Information Systems Strategic Planning. Chapter 13 in *Health Information Management: Concepts, Principles, and Practice*, 6th ed. P. Oachs and A. Watters, eds. Chicago: AHIMA.

AHIMA. 2010. RFI/RFP Template (Updated). http://library.ahima.org/xpedio/groups/public/documents/ahima/bok1_047959.hcsp?dDocName=bok1_047959.

Revoir, R. 2020. Financial Management. Chapter 25 in *Health Information Management: Concepts, Principles, and Practice*, 6th ed. P. Oachs and A Watters, eds. Chicago: AHIMA.

6.35 Clinical documentation improvement training

Competency VI.9

A clinical documentation improvement (CDI) program has been up and running for six months. Initial training of the CDI staff covered the following:

- Overview of the CDI program and goals
- MS-DRGs including CCs and MCCs and their impact on MS-DRG assignment
- The top 10 MS-DRGs for the organization
- What documentation is used for code assignment and where to find it in the paper and electronic record
- Review of clinical indicators for specific diagnosis such as respiratory failure and protein calorie malnutrition

1. After reviewing the training program, recommend four additional topics that should be covered.

2. Why are these topics important to the CDI program?

Resources

Bryant, G., S. Burgess, and M. Conroy, et al. 2013. Recruitment, selection, and orientation for CDI specialists. *Journal of AHIMA* 84(7):58–62 [expanded web version].

Patena, K. 2020. Employee Training and Development. Chapter 24 in *Health Information Management: Concepts, Principles, and Practice*, 6th ed. P. Oachs and A. Watters, eds. Chicago: AHIMA.

Prater, V. S. 2020. Human Resources Management and Professional Development. Chapter 20 in *Health Information Management Technology: An Applied Approach*, 6th ed. N. B. Sayles and L. Gordon, eds. Chicago: AHIMA.

6.36 Management principles

A

B

G

Competency VI.2

As HIM director, you have decided to bring the release of information services back in-house. For the last two years, you have outsourced that work, but continual complaints and an increasing backlog have made a change necessary.

List the managerial functions that will be necessary as you tackle this process and select at least one tool that will be used in each function. Be sure to justify the selection of the tool.

Resources

Gordon, L. 2020. Management. Chapter 17 in *Health Information Management Technology: An Applied Approach*, 6th ed. N. B. Sayles and L. Gordon, eds. Chicago: AHIMA.

Swenson, D. X. 2020. Managing and Leading During Organizational Change. Chapter 21 in *Health Information Management: Concepts, Principles, and Practice*, 6th ed. P. Oachs and A. Watters, eds. Chicago: AHIMA.

6.37 Project—contract management

Competency VI.1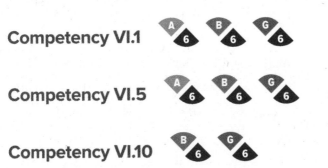

Competency VI.5

Competency VI.10

1. As HIM director, you are in charge of purchasing an encoder for your 20 coders. You have identified the criteria that you will use to make the determination and put it in the grid below. Based on this information from the requests for proposal choose an encoder vendor and justify your choice.

Type of Encoder	Vendor 1 Knowledge-based	Vendor 2 Logic-based	Vendor 3 Knowledge-based
Grouping and Pricing:			
DRG	X	X	X
APC	X	X	X
ASC	X	X	
Integrated coding references	X	X	X
Built in code edits	X	X	X
Productivity reports	X	X	
Platform	Installed	Either	Web-based
Support:			
Technical	X	X	X six months free, $500 per month after first six months
Coding		X	
Cost	$25,000 initial cost, additional $1,000 per user over 10	32,000 initial cost, additional $500.00 per user over 10	$17,500 initial cost, additional $500 per user over 10
Annual Maintenance	$5,000.00 annually	10% of total cost annually	$2,500.00 annually

2. The IT department, which was not part of the selection process, has found out that you are closing the deal on the new encoder. They ask about the interfaces between the EHR and the encoder. You realize that this is a key area that you forgot to address and learn that it is an additional cost of $2,500.00. Design a negotiation strategy to attempt to reduce or eliminate this cost.

Resources

Oachs, P. 2020. Work Design and Process Improvement. Chapter 24 in *Health Information Management: Concepts, Principles, and Practice*, 6th ed. P. Oachs and A. Watters, eds. Chicago: AHIMA.

Olson, B. D. 2020. Project Management. Chapter 26 in *Health Information Management: Concepts, Principles, and Practice*, 6th ed. P. Oachs and A. Watters, eds. Chicago: AHIMA.

6.38 Vendor contracts

Competency VI.1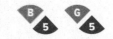

You are the coding manager for Pine Valley Regional Hospital and are in negotiations to out-source some of your coding. The vendor has drawn up a contract for your approval.

1. Review the remote coding contract that follows and determine the one significant area that has not been addressed.

2. Recommend language to insert into the contract to correct the omission.

AGREEMENT FOR REMOTE CODING SERVICES

THIS AGREEMENT made on the date and year indicated below, between **DAWSON & ASSOCIATES, LLC** (hereinafter referred to as "Contractor") and **Pine Valley Regional Hospital (PVRH)** ("Client");

WHEREAS, Client desires the services of remote coding of its Medicare, Medicaid, and commercial payor assigned charts that are scanned or made available to coders; and WHEREAS, Contractor desires to provide the service of remote coding; NOW, THEREFORE, in consideration of the mutual promises made herein and for other good and valuable consideration, it is hereby agreed by and between the parties as follows:

1. Contractor shall provide remote coding services.

    a) The Contractor understands and agrees to provide all information necessary to set up a Contract coder in the PVRH systems. This may include personal information about the contract coder including DOB, last four digits of their social security number, phone number and address in order for remote access to be added.

    b) Contract coders with 3M Coding and Reimbursement encoder and Meditech software will be sought.

    c) Contract coders will abide by the Official Coding and Reporting Guidelines, coding advice published in Coding Clinic for ICD-10-CM, CPT Assistant, except in the instance of unique payor requirements. Contract coders will also abide by PVRH coding policies and procedures.

    d) Contractor must provide proof of current coding credentials—RHIT and or CCS or CCA required with at least 1 year experience in acute care setting in either inpatient or ambulatory surgery coding.

2. In consideration of the above service, Client shall pay to Contractor the sum of FIFTY DOLLARS PER HOUR ($50):

3. Contractor will review any new contract coder provided to an PVRH facility. Contractor shall provide bi-annual quality reviews on remote coding staff at no charge to Client. At least twenty (20) records will be reviewed for each staff member per bi-annual audit.

    e) Contractor will review the first fifty (50) records of any new contract coder that is assigned to PVRH at no charge to the Client. The review results will be shared with PVRH.

f) Results of bi-annual review will be shared with Client by November 1 of every year.

g) Results of 95% for DRG assignment or less than 95% for ICD-10-CM Coding or CPT Coding a performance improvement action plan will be initiated consisting of 5% random reviews every week until quality goals are met.

4. Contractor agrees to lock in pricing with minimal increases (less than 3% increase per hourly rate) for the next 3 years.

5. Client agrees to pay Contractor the full amount of the invoice with thirty (30) days of receipt of the invoice. A service charge of one and one-half percent (1.5%) per month shall be charged for any invoices not paid within thirty (30) days of delivery of said invoice.

6. Client shall make available to Contractor at Client's expense, the means by which the Contractor can access the Client's records and Clients computer network including. (Delete - any and all hardware and software necessary including a secure ID card for Contractor to access any of Client's records and access to Client's computer network.)

   a. Contractor will be required to support their staff set up for remote access. In addition the company must provide:

      i) Adequate equipment for their contracting staff that can support remote coding

      ii) Connectivity to internet

7. Contractor is at all times acting and performing as an independent contractor and is not and shall not be deemed to be an employee of Client for any purpose whatsoever. Contractor has the full power over the determination of the hours to be worked and method of completing Contractor's responsibilities hereunder. As an independent contractor, Contractor will not receive workers' compensation, unemployment compensation, or any other fringe benefit which normally accrue to employees of Client and is responsible for providing Contractor's own benefits and paying all income withholding taxes, including FICA.

8. Upon termination of this Agreement, each party shall promptly return to the other all data, materials, and other property of the other held by it.

9. Client agrees that any and all intellectual property including copies thereof used by Contractor to perform its services are and shall remain the exclusive property of Contractor and may not be used by Client for any purpose not specifically authorized by Contractor. Intellectual property shall include, but is not limited to, processes, computer software, and educational materials.

10. Both parties will indemnify and hold the other party harmless against any liabilities, damages, and expenses including reasonable attorney fees resulting from any third-party claim or suit arising from Contractor's performance under this Agreement.

11. All notices and communications in connection with this Agreement shall be in writing and shall be considered given when delivered personally to the recipient's address as stated in this Agreement or when sent by fax to the last fax number of the recipient known to the person giving notice.

12. Either party may terminate this Agreement at any time by giving the other written notice of termination. Such notice of termination shall be effective thirty (30) days after notice is delivered. Contractor shall be responsible for carrying out all duties that have been scheduled within that thirty (30)-day termination period and Client shall be responsible for full payment of all services scheduled and performed prior to the actual date of termination.

13. This Agreement shall be governed by the laws of the State of Ohio.

14. This is the entire agreement between the parties with respect to this matter.

15. This Agreement may not be changed except in writing and signed by authorized representatives of both parties.

CLIENT: **Pine Valley Regional Hospital**

By: _____

_____

[Type or print name]

Address: _____

_____

Its: _____

Date: _____

CONTRACTOR: DAWSON & ASSOCIATES, LLC

By: _____

_____

[Type or print name]

Address: _____

_____

Its: _____

Date: _____

Source of contract Dee Mandley and Associates. Adapted and reprinted with permission.

Resource

Oachs, P. 2020. Work Design and Process Improvement. Chapter 25 in *Health Information Management: Concepts, Principles, and Practice*, 6th ed. P. Oachs and A. Watters, eds. Chicago: AHIMA.

6.39 Project management—Gantt chart

Competency VI.10

As coding manager, you are in charge of a new encoder purchase. This is your first attempt at project management and you want to perform effectively. You create a Gantt chart to illustrate the project from vendor selection to go live.

1. Determine the baseline duration of the critical path of the project.

2. Determine the variance that causes a week's delay.

3. Determine the variance that puts the project back on track.

4. Give an opinion on whether this was a successful project implementation or not and support your position.

5. Evaluate the impact of the document completion task on the overall project.

Task Name	Baseline Duration	Baseline Start	Baseline Finish	Actual Duration	Actual Start	Actual Finish
Purchase and Installation of Encoder		**Mon 2/15/16**	**Fri 7/15/16**		**Mon 2/15/16**	**Mon 7/18/16**
Select Vendor	**55 days**	**Mon 2/15/16**	**Fri 4/29/16**	**62 days**	**Mon 2/15/16**	**Tue 5/10/16**
Create List of Vendors	10 days	Mon 2/15/16	Fri 2/26/16	10 days	Mon 2/15/16	Fri 2/26/16
Send Out Request for Proposal (RFP)	20 days	Mon 2/29/16	Fri 3/25/16	20 days	Mon 2/29/16	Fri 3/25/16
Select Vendor	20 days	Mon 3/28/16	Fri 4/22/16	20 days	Mon 3/28/16	Fri 4/22/16
Finalize Contract	**5 days**	**Mon 4/25/16**	**Fri 4/29/16**	**12 days**	**Mon 4/25/16**	**Tue 5/10/16**
Department Head Signature	2 days	Mon 4/25/16	Tue 4/26/16	2 days	Mon 4/25/16	Tue 4/26/16
CEO Signature	3 days	Wed 4/27/16	Fri 4/29/16	10 days	Wed 4/27/16	Tue 5/10/16
Complete Document Requests	**5 days**	**Mon 5/2/16**	**Fri 5/6/16**	**5 days**	**Wed 5/11/16**	**Tue 5/17/16**
List of Payers	5 days	Mon 5/2/16	Fri 5/6/16	5 days	Wed 5/11/16	Tue 5/17/16
List of Discharge Dispositions	5 days	Mon 5/2/16	Fri 5/6/16	5 days	Wed 5/11/16	Tue 5/17/16
List of Reimbursement Amounts by Payer	5 days	Mon 5/2/16	Fri 5/6/16	5 days	Wed 5/11/16	Tue 5/17/16
Build Interfaces	40 days	Mon 5/9/16	Fri 7/1/16	30 days	Wed 5/18/16	Tue 6/28/16
Installation	1 day	Mon 7/4/16	Mon 7/4/16	1 day	Wed 6/29/16	Wed 6/29/16
Testing	5 days	Tue 7/5/16	Mon 7/11/16	10 days	Thu 6/30/16	Wed 7/13/16
Training	3 days	Tue 7/12/16	Thu 7/14/16	2 days	Thu 7/14/16	Fri 7/15/16
Go Live	1 day	Fri 7/15/16	Fri 7/15/16	1 day	Mon 7/18/16	Mon 7/18/16

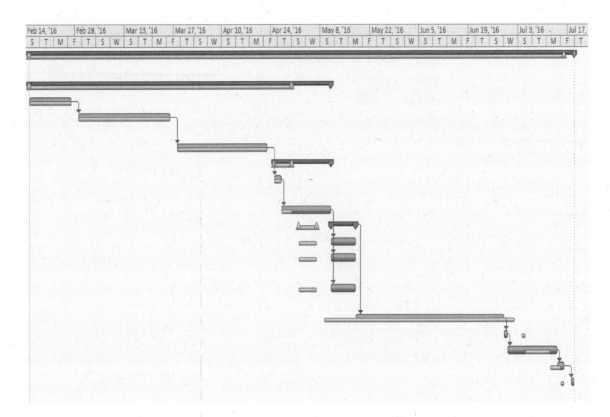

Source: GANTT chart created by M.J. Foley. Reprinted with permission.

Resource

Olson, B. D. 2020. Project Management. Chapter 26 in *Health Information Management: Concepts, Principles, and Practice*, 6th ed. P. Oachs and A. Watters, eds. Chicago: AHIMA.

6.40 Performance improvement tools

Competency VI.4

Select the most appropriate performance improvement (PI) tool or technique for each scenario below.

1. A HIM performance improvement committee wants to determine the priorities in addressing the project at hand.

2. Administration has requested a chart showing the processes changes that have been achieved from January to June.

3. A revenue cycle PI team wants to illustrate the percent of denials that are a result of a registration error.

4. A PI team wants to display data that will show if there are uncommon variations in the process.

Resource

Shaw, P. L. and D. Carter. 2019. *Quality and Performance Improvement in Healthcare: A Tool for Programmed Learning*, 7th ed. Chicago: AHIMA.

6.41 Data collection methods

Competency VI.4

You have just been hired as a coding supervisor at a local hospital. The coding department has many issues, including a two-week backlog of coding, a DNFB of over $7.5 million, and over 50 unanswered physician queries. Describe how you can use the three different data collection tools (interview, survey tools, and direct observation) to capture data that can help you improve the coding process.

Resources

Houser, S. 2020. Research methods. Chapter 18 in *Health Information Management: Concepts, Principles, and Practice*, 6th ed. P. Oachs and A. Watters, eds. Chicago: AHIMA.

Shaw, P. L. and D. Carter. 2019. *Quality and Performance Improvement in Healthcare: A Tool for Programmed Learning*, 7th ed. Chicago: AHIMA.

6.42 Discipline

Competency VI.3

A random audit showed that one of the scanner techs was not following the proper procedure for entering late records. You discussed this with him and gave him a verbal warning. Per protocol, you monitored that scanner's handling of late records for a month and found several more instances of records incorrectly processed. This time, the scanner received a written warning. How will you handle a third occurrence of this issue?

Resources

LeBlanc, M. M. 2020. Human Resources Management. Chapter 22 in *Health Information Management: Concepts, Principles, and Practice*, 6th ed. P. Oachs and A. Watters, eds. Chicago: AHIMA.

Prater, V. S. 2020. Human Resources Management and Professional Development. Chapter 20 in *Health Information Management Technology: An Applied Approach*, 6th ed. N. B. Sayles and L. Gordon, eds. Chicago: AHIMA.

6.43 Budgets

Competency VI.5

Consider that you are going to be the HIM director for a large physician group that is just organizing its practice. You are going to oversee transcription, coding, release of information, along with the other day-to-day functions of HIM. The group is planning to utilize electronic records. The electronic health record system and computers will be coming from a separate IT budget. However, you need to plan a departmental and capital budget for the first year of business. What items should you list under each budget? Keep in mind that the group has decided that anything more than $500 should be on the capital budget, except payroll expenses.

Resources

Horton, L. 2017. Statistics Computed within the Health Information Management Department. Chapter 9 in *Calculating and Reporting Healthcare Statistics*, 5th ed., revised reprint. Chicago: AHIMA.

Revoir, R. 2020. Financial Management. Chapter 25 in *Health Information Management: Concepts, Principles, and Practice*, 6th ed. P. Oachs and A. Watters, eds. Chicago: AHIMA.

6.44 Payroll variance

Competency VI.5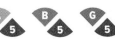

The volume of outpatient surgery and heart-center procedures has increased at your organization. Due to vacations and holidays, a significant backlog has resulted. As coding manager, you find it necessary to establish a contract with an outside vendor to reduce that backlog. Those services will be contracted for one month and payment will be at the rate of $3.50 per chart. The projected volume for the period is 365 charts per week.

At the conclusion of the vendor's service you receive this invoice.
Week 1: 377 charts coded
Week 2: 363 charts coded
Week 3: 358 charts coded
Week 4: 372 charts coded
Total: 1,470 charts coded at $3.50 per chart = $5,145.00

Classify and explain the type of budget variance depicted in this scenario.

Resource

Revoir, R. 2020. Financial Management. Chapter 25 in *Health Information Management: Concepts, Principles, and Practice*, 6th ed. P. Oachs and A. Watters, eds. Chicago: AHIMA.

6.45 Budgeting process

Competency VI.5

It is time to prepare the annual departmental operating budget for fiscal year 2019–2020. In your organization, the fiscal year runs from July 1 to June 30. At this point in time, medical records are hybrid. Build a list of at least three organizational and three departmental budget assumptions that will need clarification before the budget can be prepared.

Resources

Gordon, L. 2020. Management. Chapter 17 in *Health Information Management Technology: An Applied Approach*, 6th ed. N. B. Sayles and L. Gordon, eds. Chicago: AHIMA.

Revoir, R. 2020. Financial Management. Chapter 25 in *Health Information Management: Concepts, Principles, and Practice*, 6th ed. P. Oachs and A. Watters, eds. Chicago: AHIMA.

6.46 Cost reporting

Competency VI.5

Pine Valley Community Hospital, a critical access hospital, has hired you to be their HIM director. During your first weeks on the job, you hear the finance director talk about cost reports that are unfamiliar to you. Your previous position was manager of HIM at a small acute-care facility. You do some research to learn about the function of cost reports. You discover why you have not encountered cost reports previously during your research. Supply that rationale, while providing an analysis of cost reports and include a comparison of the four methods of allocating overhead costs.

Resources

Gordon, L. 2020. Management. Chapter 17 in *Health Information Management Technology: An Applied Approach*, 6th ed. N. B. Sayles and L. Gordon, eds. Chicago: AHIMA.

Revoir, R. 2020. Financial Management. Chapter 25 in *Health Information Management: Concepts, Principles, and Practice*, 6th ed. P. Oachs and A. Watters, eds. Chicago: AHIMA.

6.47 Budget variance

Competency VI.5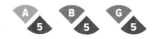

Your organization is in the process of microfilming all the old records in storage. The budget for this process is $500,000 over three years. You have contracted with a company to perform the microfilm services at $0.09 per page and have estimated that there are about 5.5 million pages to be converted. At the end of the first year, you review the invoice and see that you have been billed for converting 2,083,333 pages.

1. Determine your budget variance and what type it is.

2. Provide a short explanation that can be given to administration regarding the variance.

Resource

Revoir, R. 2020. Financial Management. Chapter 25 in *Health Information Management: Concepts, Principles, and Practice*, 6th ed. P. Oachs and A. Watters, eds. Chicago: AHIMA.

6.48 Personal health record choices

Competency VI.8

Your 70-year-old retired grandfather is very computer-literate. He also has multiple health issues and sees a number of different specialists. He recently heard about personal health records (PHRs) and would like you to explain the various options to him. Provide your grandfather with the requested information and advise him on which selection might best suit his needs.

Reference

AHIMA Personal Health Record Practice Council. 2006. Helping consumers select PHRs: questions and considerations for navigating an emerging market. *Journal of AHIMA* 77(10):50–56.

6.49 Social determinants of health

Competency VI.8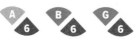

For the following scenario, identify how each of the five domains of social determinants of health (economic stability, education, health and healthcare, neighborhood and built environment, social and community context) could negatively influence the patient's healthcare outcomes.

An 86-year-old native Russian woman lives alone in an apartment on the outskirts of the city. While her husband was alive, they lived in a house in a Russian-speaking community where they both grew up after immigrating. Since his passing last year, she had to move to this tiny second floor walk-up apartment in an unfamiliar area with neighbors who speak Spanish. She has not made many friends there since she moved in ten months ago. All of her physicians and the nearest hospital are on the other side of the city, and it takes almost fifty minutes to get there. There is no bus service to that part of the city from where she lives, and she does not drive anymore. She relies on old friends to take her to medical appointments when they can, as her only child lives out of state and taxis are too expensive. She frequently misses appointments due to transportation issues or because she has confused times or places. She lives on a fixed income with Medicare and a very small pension from her husband. Her academic education is at a seventh-grade level.

1. If this patient was being seen at a provider's office where you were part of the team, propose solutions that could help mitigate at least three domain issues you identify.

2. What inferences can you draw about this patient's healthcare literacy? Provide support for your answer.

Reference

Sandefer, R. 2020. Consumer Health Informatics. Chapter 14 in *Health Information Management: Concepts, Principles, and Practice*, 6th ed. P. Oachs and A. Watters, eds. Chicago: AHIMA.

6.50 Quality management tools

Competency VI.4

Choose the appropriate quality management tool for each scenario presented below and defend your selection.

1. Your multidisciplinary performance improvement team is working on solutions to poor bed turnaround time. You have collected data on the issue and discovered there are seven main problems. Recommend the quality management tool that should be used to prioritize the problems. This tool will allow identification of the problems most responsible for the poor bed turnaround time.

2. Unfortunately, your healthcare organization has experienced a sentinel event, which is an unexpected death or serious physical injury. You will be part of the team that works on the root cause analysis. What quality management tool is most often used in this process?

3. The chief of staff is helping the HIM department reduce the number of delinquent charts. He has asked for an illustration that shows the various medical departments (orthopedics, dermatology, ophthalmology, urology, respiratory) and the percentage of the overall delinquencies for which they are responsible. What quality management tool will show this information appropriately?

4. Your performance improvement team has been tracking a key process improvement for the past year. What quality management tool will be of assistance in tracking any variances?

5. A process improvement team is collecting data to determine if there is a correlation between medication errors and pharmacy tech overtime. What is the best tool to plot this data?

References

Shaw, P. L. and D. Carter. 2019. *Quality and Performance Improvement in Healthcare, A Tool for Programmed Learning,* 7th ed. Chicago: AHIMA.

Williamson, L. M. 2020. Research and Data Analysis. Chapter 13 in *Health Information Management Technology: An Applied Approach*, 6th ed. N. B. Sayles and L. Gordon, eds. Chicago: AHIMA.

6.51 Change management

Competency VI.1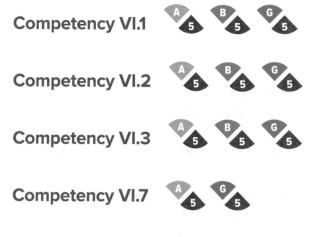

Competency VI.2

Competency VI.3

Competency VI.7

Competency VI.9

Gretchen McMasters, RHIA, is the HIM director at Maple Heights Memorial hospital. Gretchen has a meeting today with Cynthia Robinson, CCS, the lead coder. Cynthia is a very good coder and has the lead position by virtue of her years of experience.

Gretchen's meeting with Cynthia today revolves around the findings of an internal investigation, which showed that Cynthia inappropriately accessed her neighbors' patient records. She had done this on multiple occasions. Cynthia had no rebuttal, as she had no reason beyond curiosity for looking at the records. Gretchen fires Cynthia for her breach of privacy. She tells her to clear out her desk and leave the hospital now. Gretchen plans to hold a staff meeting tomorrow to address privacy breaches.

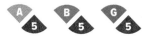

1. In the wake of this change, recommend how Gretchen should handle tomorrow's meeting. Propose aspects of privacy training that should be reviewed with the staff.

2. Refer to the previous scenario and assess Gretchen's handling of the lead coder's termination with a focus on how that interaction could have been handled in a more appropriate manner. Take into consideration aspects of risk management in your response.

3. Evaluate the ethical responsibility that Gretchen has in this situation.

References

Kelly, J. and P. Greenstone. 2016. *Management for the Health Information Professional*. Chicago: AHIMA.

LeBlanc, M. 2020. Human Resources Management. Chapter 22 in *Health Information Management: Concepts, Principles, and Practice*, 6th ed. P. Oachs and A. Watters, eds. Chicago: AHIMA.

Reynolds, R. B. and M. S. Brodnik. 2017. The HIPAA Security Rule. Chapter 12 in *Fundamentals of Law for Health Informatics and Information Management,* 3rd ed. M. S. Brodnik, L. A. Rinehart-Thompson, and R. B. Reynolds, eds. Chicago: AHIMA.

Shaw P. L. and D. Carter. 2019. *Quality and Performance Improvement in Healthcare: A Tool for Programmed Learning*, 7th ed. Chicago: AHIMA.

Swirsky, E. 2020. Ethical Issues in Health Information Management. Chapter 27 in *Health Information Management: Concepts, Principles, and Practice*, 6th ed. P. Oachs and A. Watters, eds. Chicago: AHIMA.

6.52 Disability and diversity

Competency VI.6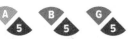

Carly, the coding supervisor at Beechwood Memorial Hospital, is in the process of hiring a new outpatient coder to join the team of four that are already on staff. She has been trying to fill the position for several months without success. This has caused the outpatient discharged not final billed (DNFB) to climb significantly and there is pressure to hire someone soon.

The new coder will train in-house for three to six months before transitioning to work from home. The current work process, in addition to coding, includes telephone attendance at weekly "huddles" to discuss immediate coding, departmental, or organizational issues that arise. Also, coders are required to be on site to attend quarterly coding meetings, and monthly coding education sessions.

Today, Carly has received an outstanding resume for an experienced outpatient coder. The candidate has previous experience with both the information system and the encoder that the hospital uses, so training should be able to be expedited. Carly's concern, however, is that the applicant is deaf. She recognizes that this will require accommodations and is unsure how the staff will react to interacting with a colleague with such a disability.

1. Assess the accommodations that may need to be implemented if a deaf coder is hired.

2. What steps might Carly take to promote diversity if she hires this applicant?

Reference

Kelly, J. and P. Greenstone. 2016. Leadership Concepts in Health Information Management. Chapter 3 in *Management for the Health Information Professional*. Chicago: AHIMA.

6.53 Electronic health record contract

Competency VI.7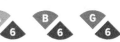

A new pediatric group, Elmhurst Pediatric Group, has been formed and you have been chosen as the information technology (IT) manager. A local hospital has reached out to the group offering participation in their electronic health record (EHR). The proposal states that the pediatric group will pay 15 percent of the hospital's costs related to the services. This seems like a good arrangement since investing in an EHR independently will require a significant capital expenditure. You speak with the IT director at the hospital and find out that the EHR is certified and interoperable. You are told that BigPharmRX is the only e-prescribing application that is permitted to be used with the EHR, but the EHR can be used for all payers. Your primary concern is that there would be a referral quota that the group would need to meet in order to secure this arrangement. However, you were assured that there are no referral strings tied to the arrangement.

You are unsure if this proposal will comply with the EHR safe harbors. Conduct an investigation and create a memo for the management team with your findings, providing supported opinions on whether or not the proposal complies with EHR safe harbor mandates.

If you determine the proposal does not meet the requirements, what aspect(s) could be modified to achieve compliance?

Reference

Bowman, S. 2017. Corporate Compliance. Chapter 18 in *Fundamentals of Law for Health Informatics and Information Management*, 3rd ed. M. S. Brodnik, L. A. Rinehart-Thompson, R. B. Reynolds, eds. Chicago: AHIMA.

6.54 Patient satisfaction scores

Competency VI.8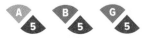

In the physician practice where you are the office manager, the providers are disappointed in their patient satisfaction scores. Feedback indicates that patients are frustrated with the amount of time it takes to schedule an appointment when they call in, commenting that the office line is often busy. However, the patients were pleased that they have the ability to view test results via the patient portal.

Recommend to the providers how the patient portal can be used beyond supplying test results in ways that might improve their satisfaction scores.

Reference

Brixey, J., S. Biederman, and D. Dolezel. 2017. Consumer Health Informatics. Chapter 15 in *Introduction to Healthcare Informatics*, 2nd ed. S. Biedermann and D. Dolezel, eds. Chicago: AHIMA.

6.55 Consumer informatics

Competency VI.8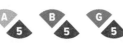

As the HIM director for Pine Valley Hospital, a small, rural critical access hospital, you are interested in promoting consumer informatics for your older patient population. Your goal is to establish a class where patients could come to learn about on-line health information. Survey data shows that a majority of your facility's patients are 60 and older and on fixed incomes. While most have internet access, few have computers; instead, they rely on tablets or smartphones. Determine the key points to cover during a class to assist end-users with consumer informatics.

Reference

Brixey, J., S. Biederman, and D. Dolezel. 2017. Consumer Health Informatics. Chapter 15 in *Introduction to Healthcare Informatics*, 2nd ed. S. Biedermann and D. Dolezel, eds. Chicago: AHIMA.

6.56 Addressing health literacy

Competency VI.8

You work in HIM at a hospital in an area that has had an influx of immigrants from India. Administration is frustrated by the overuse of the emergency department by this population. Communication with the primary care providers in the area has verified that the overall health literacy of this population is low.

1. Forecast at least four benefits that may be realized for providers if the populations' health literacy is improved.

2. Develop a plan to address the health literacy challenges of this population.

Reference

Brixey, J., S. Biederman, and D. Dolezel. 2017. Consumer Health Informatics. Chapter 15 in *Introduction to Healthcare Informatics*, 2nd ed. S. Biedermann and D. Dolezel, eds. Chicago: AHIMA.

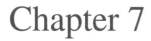

Chapter 7

Extended Cases

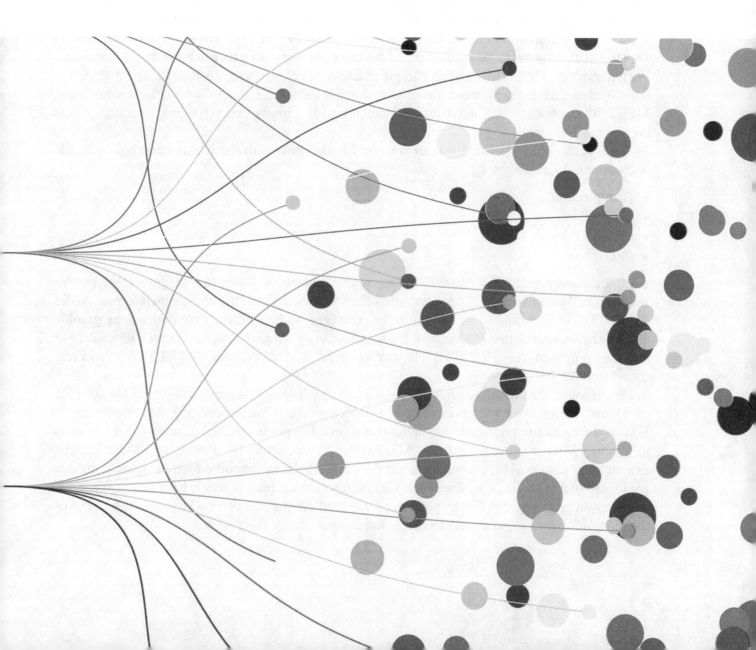

7.0 Multiple patient admissions

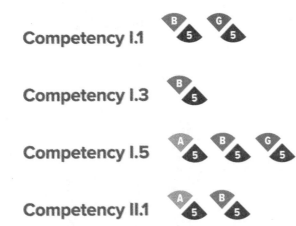

Competency I.1

Competency I.3

Competency I.5

Competency II.1

A 72-year-old male came to the emergency room with a severe headache. As this was his first visit at St. Stephen's Hospital, all of his information had to be entered in the electronic health record including his name, David L. Smythe; his date of birth 9/02/1948; his insurance, Medicare; and his social security number 971-26-6798. Mr. Smythe was assigned medical record number 405589, and his account number for the visit was H647191. His blood pressure was elevated at 185/102 with hypertensive urgency noted by the physician, who then administered Lisinopril. Within minutes, Mr. Smythe had an allergic reaction (urticaria) to the Lisinopril. The medication was discontinued and the patient was observed in ER for several hours. The headache abated and Mr. Smythe was sent home and instructed to contact his primary care physician for control of his high blood pressure.

Three weeks later, Mr. Smythe returns to the ER, this time with significant chest pain. The ER doctor ran the following tests:

- Troponin level
- CPK
- CKMB
- EKG

All indications pointed to a non-STEMI myocardial infarction. With that diagnosis, the patient was admitted to the hospital. The registration clerk who completed the admission information did not find David L. Smith's information in the computer, so he entered Mr. Smith's demographic and insurance information (Medicare); his social security number 171-26-6789; DOB 9/02/1948 and the admission date (7/1/2020). He was assigned account number H647302 under medical record number 612392.

Per protocol, the attending physician started the patient on Lisinopril, to which Mr. Smythe developed severe angioedema evidenced by significant lip and tongue swelling, and throat itching. Benadryl was administered and the swelling subsided. The physician then changed the medication to Vasotec without subsequent issue. Meanwhile, a request had been made that a cardiologist examine the patient. The examination led the cardiologist to schedule an immediate coronary angiography that was delayed due to the allergic reaction the patient was experiencing. When the coronary angiography was finally performed, the cardiologist identified a 90 percent blockage of the circumflex artery and inserted a drug-eluting stent.

The next day, the patient complained of shortness of breath, and a chest x-ray was completed, which indicated a suspicious mass in the lower right lobe. A CT scan of the chest and abdomen was performed, confirming the large mass with additional concerns for lesions in the liver. Upon conferring, a pulmonologist recommended percutaneous lung and liver biopsies. An interventional radiologist performed both biopsy procedures with the pathology report indicating adenocarcinoma of the right lower lobe and metastatic adenocarcinoma to the liver, which was noted in the patient's discharge summary. An oncologist weighed in on the plan of care for newly diagnosed cancer and requested that a dietician assess the patient, as his BMI of 22.31 indicated a moderate protein calorie malnutrition.

The day before the patient was to be discharged, he fell and sustained a severely displaced left radial styloid fracture. The patient was taken to surgery under the care of the orthopaedist and underwent an open reduction and internal fixation of the closed fracture.

A month after discharge, a request for Mr. Smythe's records is received in the health information management (HIM) department from Mr. Smythe's daughter. She wants copies of Mr. Smythe's records sent to an attorney.

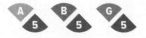

1. Determine the appropriate ICD-10-CM code(s) as appropriate for Mr. Smythe's initial emergency room visit.

2. An error occurred with Mr. Smythe's accounts. Determine the issue and department responsible for the error. Additionally, determine the impact this error had on the patient's care. Recommend options that could reduce the likelihood of this type of issue occurring in the future.

3. Consider the request for Mr. Smythe's personal health records and develop a reasoned response on whether to release the records or not.

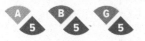

4. Assess the mapping of these ICD-10-CM cancer codes to the ICD-O-3 code supplied. If you identify an error(s), determine what correction should be made.

ICD-10-CM code	ICD-O-3 code
C34.31	8140/6
C78.7	8140/3

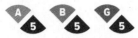

5. Differentiate RxNorm's concept unique identifier (RxCUI) from its corresponding NDC number for Lisinopril. Assume that the Lisinopril was dosed as a 40mg. oral tablet (from a 30-count bottle) from Aidarex Pharmaceuticals. Use RxNorm's semantic clinical drug term type.

References

Giannangelo, K. 2019. *Healthcare Code Sets, Clinical Terminologies, and Classification Systems*, 4th ed. Chicago: AHIMA.

Morey, A. and R. B. Reynolds. 2020. Health Record Content and Documentation. Chapter 4 in *Health Information Management: Concepts, Principles, and Practice*, 6th ed. P. Oachs and A. Watters, eds. Chicago: AHIMA.

NDC List. 2019. https://ndclist.com/?s=lisinopril.

Rinehart-Thompson, L. A. 2017. HIPAA Privacy Rule: Part 1. Chapter 10 in *Fundamentals of Law for Health Informatics and Information Management,* 3rd ed. M. S. Brodnik, L. A. Rinehart-Thompson, and R. B. Reynolds, eds. Chicago: AHIMA.

RxNorm. 2019. https://mor.nlm.nih.gov/RxNav/search?searchBy=RXCUI&searchTerm=197884.

Sayles, N. B. 2020. Health Information Functions, Purpose, and Users. Chapter 3 in *Health Information Management Technology: An Applied Approach*, 6th ed. N. B. Sayles and L. Gordon, eds. Chicago: AHIMA.

7.1 A day in the life of an HIM director

Competency I.2

Competency I.6

Competency II.1

Competency III.3

Competency III.4

Competency IV.2

Competency IV.3

Competency V.1

Competency V.2

Competency VI.3

Laura Oliver is the HIM director for Cedar Hills Psychiatric Hospital, located in Columbus, Ohio. She has 15 years of experience in HIM with five of them as a director. Here is a typical day in her work life at this licensed by the state of Ohio, 200 bed, Medicare-participating facility.

7:45 a.m. While at home preparing to testify at court later this morning, Laura fields a phone call from a concerned release of information (ROI) clerk. The clerk has a police officer in her office requesting the blood type and physical characteristics of a woman who has been a former patient at the facility. The ROI clerk refused to release the information but the officer was insistent. Laura asks to speak directly to the police officer, who explains that the requested information is needed to help locate a paranoid schizophrenic woman who is missing from a group home.

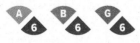

1. Conduct an assessment as to Laura's obligation to fulfill this request. Supply relevant legal corroboration to support your position.

8:37 a.m.   While waiting to be called to testify in the court proceeding, Laura works on a request from human resources to supply information needed for a new position in her department, that of Clinical Documentation Improvement Specialist. Human resources asked for education requirements, job experience, and the skills necessary for the position.

2. Propose the qualifications necessary for this job to provide to human resources.

9:33 a.m.   Ms. Oliver has a new employee who is responsible for collecting information for reporting to the Ohio Trauma Registry as necessary. This is Betty's first day and she is lost on one of the first data elements to be collected: the hospital code.

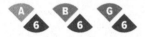

3. According to the Ohio Trauma Registry data dictionary, a four-digit code represents the hospital. How should Laura advise Betty to determine the code for the hospital? What is the code that Betty should use?

10:18 a.m.   Ms. Oliver is called to the witness stand in a case of alleged malpractice against a staff psychiatrist. She was asked to bring the patient record from his 8/31/19 admission, which ended with the patient's death on 10/2/19.

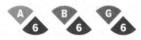

4. Formulate appropriate responses by Ms. Oliver to the questions below as she attempts to comply with the legal process and provide support for those decisions.
    a) How long have you been in your position as HIM director and custodian of health records?

    b) Was this record prepared in the normal course of business?

    c) Can you read the progress note dated 10/01/2019?

    d) In your opinion, was the delay in ordering a chest x-ray warranted?

    e) There is an ER record from a transferring facility that was supplied with the documents as it was used in decision making for the patient. The attorney wants to know if this was created in the normal course of business.

12:01 p.m.   Laura begins preparation for the quarterly Medical Records Committee meeting with the medical staff next week. The committee Chairman inquiring as to the legitimacy of texting patient orders forwarded that question as an agenda item to Laura.

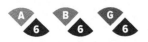

5. Develop an appropriate medical staff policy to propose to the committee based on research. Imagine there will be pushback on the recommendation. Prepare three talking points that communicate sound rationale in support of the recommendation.

1:15 p.m.   Ms. Oliver meets with Matilda, a scanner tech in the HIM department. The reason for the meeting is that Matilda, a long-time, conscientious employee, has recently begun having an increasing number of issues. She has been late to work on two occasions this past month, which the department supervisor addressed with her in a one-on-one meeting. Now, she is scanning records to the wrong patient medical record accounts, and her workload is falling behind. Matilda explains that she has been distracted at work because her youngest son has been having issues in school related to bullying. Laura is sympathetic to Matilda's family situation and would like to be lenient in applying disciplinary action. She calls Charles, the HR director, to get his input before making a decision. During a conversation with Charles, Laura is reminded that Cedar Hill's HR policies for disciplinary action follow a progressive penalty approach: verbal warning, written warning, suspension, and termination.

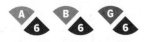

6. Propose the disciplinary action, if any, that Ms. Oliver should dispense to Matilda with justification in order to meet human resource's requirements. Theorize what argument Charles used to help Laura arrive at her decision.

2:03 p.m.   Laura receives a call from the ER charge nurse. She has a concern about an uninsured patient who arrived in a private car after being directed by the triage nurse at Oak Ridge Memorial Hospital emergency room (part of the 250 bed, state of Ohio licensed, Medicare-participating hospital) to come to Cedar Hills for care. Cedar Hill's ER doctor found the patient to be severely depressed with suicidal ideations and promptly admitted him. The ER charge nurse thinks that Oak Ridge Memorial violated the law and wants Laura's opinion.

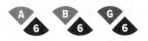

7. Identify the law that applies to this situation and provide an opinion regarding whether or not the law was violated by Oak Ridge Memorial Hospital and support your position.

3:00 p.m.   Meeting with the Chief Financial Officer (CFO) on the discharged not final billed (DNFB) report. Ms. Oliver has prepared a data display for the DNFB for the past ten weeks with the data below.

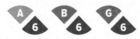

8. Create an appropriate data display for the data. Suppose that today is the third Tuesday of January. Hypothesize on the explanation that Ms. Oliver will give as explanation for the recent trend evidenced by the data. What is the most likely reason for the 12/2/19 spike in the DNFB?

11/18/19	$652,014.23
11/25/19	$679,336.45
12/2/19	$845,278.61
12/9/19	$791,699.07
12/16/19	$792,466.36
12/23/19	$795,844.83
12/30/19	$1,017,659.22
1/6/20	$1,188,571.98
1/13/20	$998,475.36
1/20/20	$787,494.80

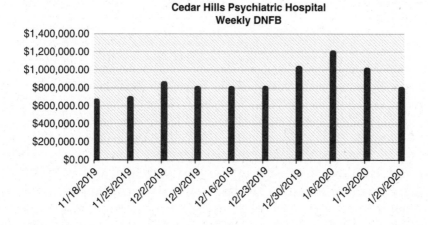

3:42 p.m. Laura receives a telephone call from a harried new staff psychiatrist. Dr. Fleming is calling from her personal office, where she has just seen a patient who was threatening his ex-wife (Julia Goodwin) with bodily harm. Dr. Fleming believes the threat to be legitimate and wants to alert the ex-wife to the threat but she is concerned that her communication of that information would be a violation of the HIPAA Privacy Rule.

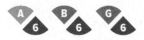

9. Formulate a response to Dr. Fleming addressing her HIPAA concern and indicate whether or not Dr. Fleming should contact Ms. Goodwin. Provide relevant supporting legal doctrine for the basis of your response.

4:45 p.m. After addressing Dr. Fleming's concerns, Laura leaves the office knowing that tomorrow will bring a new set of questions and problems that will need to be addressed.

References

AHIMA. 2014. Clinical Documentation Improvement Toolkit. Chicago: AHIMA.

Brodnik, M. S. 2017. Access, Use, and Disclosure and Release of Health Information. Chapter 15 in *Fundamentals of Law for Health Informatics and Information Management,* 3rd ed. M. S. Brodnik, L. A. Rinehart-Thompson, and R. B. Reynolds, eds. Chicago: AHIMA.

Brodnik, M. S., L. A. Rinehart-Thompson, and R. B. Reynolds. 2017. HIPAA Privacy Rule: Part I. Chapter 10 in *Fundamentals of Law for Health Informatics and Information Management,* 3rd ed. Chicago: AHIMA.

Centers for Medicare and Medicaid (CMS). 2019. Texting of Patient Information among Healthcare Providers. https://www.cms.gov/Medicare/Provider-Enrollment-and-Certification /SurveyCertificationGenInfo/Downloads/Survey-and-Cert-Letter-18-10.pdf.

Joint Commission. n.d. Texting—Use of Secure Text Messaging for Patient Orders. Accessed August 22, 2019. https://www.jointcommission.org/standards_information/jcfaqdetails.aspx?StandardsFAQId=1 616&StandardsFAQChapterId=23&ProgramId=0&ChapterId=0&IsFeatured=False&IsNew=False& Keyword=.

Joint Commission. 2016. Clarification: Use of Secure Text Messaging for Patient Care Orders is Not Acceptable. https://www.jointcommission.org/assets/1/6/Clarification_Use_of_Secure_Text _Messaging.pdf.

Ohio Department of Public Safety. 2019a. Ohio Trauma Registry 2019 Trauma Acute Care Registry Data Dictionary. https://www.publicsafety.ohio.gov/links/ems_OTR-TACR-Data-Dictionary-2019.pdf.

Ohio Department of Public Safety. 2019b. Hospital Code List. http://www.publicsafety.ohio.gov/links /EMS_DC_FacilityCodes.xlsx.

Prater, V. S. 2020. Human Resources Management and Professional Development. Chapter 20 in *Health Information Management Technology: An Applied Approach*, 6th ed. N. B. Sayles and L. Gordon, eds. Chicago: AHIMA.

Rinehart-Thompson, L. A. 2017a. Legal Proceedings. Chapter 4 in *Fundamentals of Law for Health Informatics and Information Management,* 3rd ed. M. S. Brodnik, L. A. Rinehart-Thompson, and R. B. Reynolds, eds. Chicago: AHIMA.

Rinehart-Thompson, L. A. 2017b. Patient Rights and Responsibilities. Chapter 14 in *Fundamentals of Law for Health Informatics and Information Management,* 3rd ed. M. S. Brodnik, L. A. Rinehart-Thompson, and R. B. Reynolds, eds. Chicago: AHIMA.

7.2 Coding productivity process

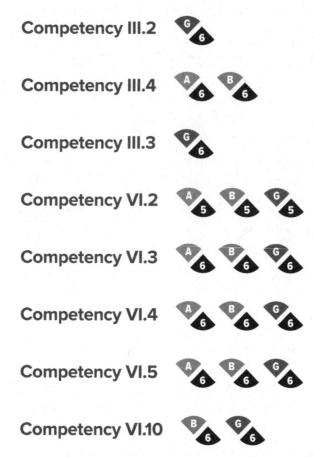

Competency III.2

Competency III.4

Competency III.3

Competency VI.2

Competency VI.3

Competency VI.4

Competency VI.5

Competency VI.10

Aspen Hills Hospital's HIM director, Sabrina Cavanaugh is meeting with her coding supervisor, Patricia Reynolds, who has been concerned about inpatient coding productivity. Since ICD-10 implementation, productivity numbers have fallen and never rebounded like Patricia expected they would as coders became more familiar with the new classification system. Outsourcing costs as well as the discharged not final billed (DNFB) totals have been rising. There is pressure from administration to lower or eliminate the costs associated with outsourcing altogether. Currently, the outsourcing productivity standard is two charts per hour and rate of pay is $35.00 per hour. Inpatient discharges are relatively stable pre- and post-ICD-10 implementation, running between 60 to 70 discharges per day. Prior to ICD-10, there was no outsourcing, with seasonal increases in discharge volumes handled by overtime.

The following are coding staff details; productivity is calculated per hour.

Experience	Age	Credential	Records	Coder	Coding Quality	Goal Productivity Prior	Productivity Prior to ICD-10	Goal Productivity Post	Productivity Post ICD-10
30	61	CCS	Inpatient	Kathy Miller	97%	3	3.5	3	1.9
16	48	RHIT	Inpatient	John Reeves	95%	3	3.1	3	1.5
7	33		Inpatient	Charles Hathaway	94%	3	2.9	3	1.25
20	42	CCS	Outpatient/ER	Leonard Lobmiller	96%	15	17	15	16
2	24		Outpatient/ER	Jessica McCarthy	93%	15	18	15	17
10	37	RHIT	Outpatient/OPS	Andrea Delaware	94%	6	6.5	6	6
5	28	CCA	Outpatient/ANC	Carmella Casetti	95%	30	35	30	35
14	50		Outpatient/ANC	Robert Neff	92%	30	29	30	30

The full coding staff receive monthly education and, in general, have very good coding quality scores. All credentialed coders maintain their certifications with CEUs from various webinars and seminars they attend. The group works remotely, but technology is challenging for Kathy, Robert, and Charles. They often have to call IT for support with issues that the other coders can troubleshoot themselves. This has strained the relationship between IT and HIM. IT sometimes must spend a significant amount of time fixing issues for the remote coders. Coders feel that IT staff do not recognize the importance of coding to the bottom line of the hospital, especially when their requests for help are not answered in a timely manner or taken seriously.

Inpatient and outpatient coders are not cross-trained, but all outpatient coders can code all varieties of outpatient records, including ancillary accounts, ERs, outpatient surgeries, and observations. There is little cohesiveness between the inpatient and outpatient coders.

There has been little turnover in the coding staff, but one coder is approaching retirement, and another was hired just two years ago, right out of college. They have 30 and 2 years of experience respectively, while the other coders average 12 years of experience.

Coding staff are insistent that the current productivity standards are unreasonable. One of the things they take issue with is that the standards are built on the assumption of a full 8 hours a day spent coding. Staff know that they spend time throughout their day on other activities not just coding.

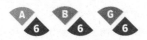

1. One of the first things that Sabrina asks Patricia to do is a work measurement study. Using the information below, finish building the table and propose a new standard for inpatient productive time (round to whole number). All three coders worked 80 hours in this two-week period for the work-study.

Inpatient Minutes per Week on Tasks						
Week One	Telephone Calls	Denials	Querying	Email	Coding	Lunch
Kathy Miller	100	175	100	45		30
John Reeves	75	75	50	45		30
Charles Hathaway	75	75	50	45		30
Week Two						
Kathy Miller	90	125	125	50		30
John Reeves	80	60	60	45		30
Charles Hathaway	60	50	60	55		30

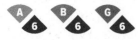

2. Using the coding staff data supplied previously, create a bar graph to illustrate the pre and post-ICD-10 implementation productivity for both individual inpatient coders and for the inpatient coding team as a whole.

Patricia thinks implementing a computer-assisted coding (CAC) program might help with the productivity issues. She is aware that the number of CAC vendors has grown over the past three years, including 3M, Optum, and others. In her research, she finds that the CAC software may need a specific interface in order to function. In addition, the cost of CAC software varies depending on the information system to which it must tie in and the number of users of the application. Trained coders should be used in conjunction with a CAC program to review the proposed codes and make a determination on their appropriateness. Vendors claim that some of the cost of a CAC can be recouped with savings achieved through increased coder productivity. Patricia's investigation shows that increases in coder productivity can range from 20 to 35 percent. The requests for proposal have identified one vendor that stands out. The entire cost of the implementation would be $80,000, and they are standing behind a 25 percent productivity increase. Additional benefits may be realized in reduction of time spend on denials and queries and an increase in the case-mix index.

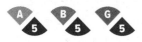

3. Create a SWOT analysis regarding the purchase of a CAC application.

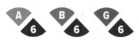

4. Based on the time study results for actual time that inpatient coders spend coding, present the figures for the number of charts coded daily and biweekly for the coding team overall. Be sure to present the numbers for pre and post ICD-10 implementation as well as if a 25 percent productivity increase was realized with a CAC implementation. Provide calculations to nearest whole number. Then forecast the annual savings on outsourcing expenditures that would occur with a 25 percent productivity increase.

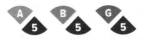

5. Sabrina knows that the organization requires at least a 33 percent return on investment for major purchases such as CAC software. Compile the data necessary to arrive at the return on investment and forecast if Sabrina will be able to receive the necessary funds for the purchase.

6. Create a GANTT chart to manage the project based on the following information.

The decision was made to proceed with the CAC implementation and Sabrina delegated the management of this project to Patricia. Patricia recognized the importance of balancing a smooth implementation process with the need to get this project completed in a quick manner. Therefore, she developed an aggressive timeline for the project from the contract through the go-live scheduled for 2/24/20.

The kick-off for the project will begin with the contract completion process. At Aspen Hills, the department director and the CEO must both sign off on the contract. Patricia sets the start date as 1/20/2020. She allows 3 days for Sabrina to sign the contract, and another 8 days for the CEO, Judith Adler to sign and return the contract. Unfortunately, Sabrina has the flu the week the contract is to be signed and does not come in to work. On Thursday, 1/23/2020, she calls Patricia to touch base and realizes that the project is going to be a week behind schedule if she does not sign the contract until she returns to work next week. She has Patricia fax her the contract, which she immediately signs and faxes back. Patricia sends the contract to the CEO the next day and gets it back one day sooner than the originally planned date of 1/30/2020. On 1/30/2020, the signed contract is sent to the vendor for signatures, which Patricia had originally allowed to be completed by 2/5/2020 but actually took until 2/7/2020.

When Patricia realized the contract was not going to be finished on time, she needed to reschedule the installation of the software, which had been planned for 2/7/2020. This had to be pushed back a week, until 2/14/2020, because of the vendor's other commitments.

Similarly, the testing phase was rescheduled as well, moving from 2/10 through 2/11 to 2/15 through 2/16. Since Patricia was responsible for the testing phase, she decided to work over the weekend to help move the project closer to being on track.

Patricia decided that in addition to herself, they would train one inpatient and one outpatient coder as super users. She chose the most experienced coder from each group who were technology savvy to train. She originally allotted three days for this training, from 2/12 through 2/14. As it turned out, the training had to be delayed to a 2/17 start date because the installation and testing ran over. Luckily, the vendor was able to accommodate her request. Their super user training finished a day earlier than planned as they all caught on very quickly to the use of the software. By virtue of the ease of use of the software, Patricia felt that the rest of the coders could be trained in three days instead of five as originally planned. Therefore, the training could be moved from 2/17 through 2/21 to 2/19 through 2/21, thus preserving the go-live date of 2/24, which went off without a hitch.

References

Horton, L. A. 2017. *Calculating and Reporting Healthcare Statistics,* 5th ed. revised reprint. Chicago: AHIMA.

Kelly, J. and P. Greenstone. 2016. *Management for the Health Information Professional*. Chicago: AHIMA.

Marc, D. 2020. Data Visualization. Chapter 17 in *Health Information Management: Concepts, Principles, and Practice*, 6th ed. P. Oachs and A. Watters, eds. Chicago: AHIMA.

Oachs, P. 2020. Work Design and Process Improvement. Chapter 25 in *Health Information Management: Concepts, Principles, and Practice*, 6th ed. P. Oachs and A. Watters, eds. Chicago: AHIMA.

7.3 Missing laptop

Scenario 1

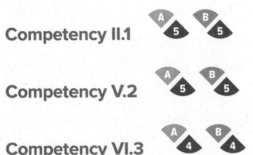

Competency II.1

Competency V.2

Competency VI.3

Gertrude, a home health nurse for New Horizons Hospital, accidentally left her encrypted laptop at the home of her client, Mr. Morgan. She noticed it was missing when she arrived at the next and last client of the day's residence. The laptop had access to information about all home health clients, including visit notes, medications, and demographic and payment information. She immediately rescheduled that appointment and backtracked to retrieve the laptop, but when she arrived at Mr. Morgan's home forty minutes after originally departing, no one was there. Then she remembered Mr. Morgan mentioned a doctor's appointment that afternoon. She called the home health office to request Mr. Morgan's cell phone number. When she reached him 10 minutes later, Mr. Morgan stated he had the laptop with him and would leave it with the receptionist at the podiatrist's office for her to pick up. Gertrude tried to ask where he was but he interrupted saying Judy just called him back to the exam room and he had to go, hanging up. Gertrude began calling every local podiatrist asking if someone named Judy worked there, hoping to establish where the laptop was. Finally, after 35 minutes of calling, she found the right office. She explained the situation to Judy, who said she had the laptop and Gertrude could come by anytime tomorrow to get it. The office was closing since it was 4:00 p.m. and no one was able to stay for her to come by that evening. When the office opened at 8:00 a.m. the next morning, Gertrude was there to retrieve the laptop. Unfortunately, the laptop was nowhere to be found. It was surmised that perhaps someone from the cleaning crew that worked the night before may have taken the laptop, as nothing else was missing from the office. Gertrude left to go report the theft to her manager.

1. Formulate a plan of action that the home health manager should initiate detailing the steps.

2. Propose appropriate disciplinary action (if any) for Gertrude.

3. Construct a list of internal and external individuals who need to be notified of this theft and provide a rationale for their inclusion.

Scenario 2

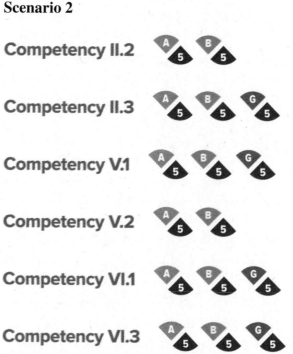

Competency II.2

Competency II.3

Competency V.1

Competency V.2

Competency VI.1

Competency VI.3

Walnut Grove Hospital outsources some inpatient coding to Waldorf and Associates, with whom they have a business associate agreement. Eloise Apple is an independent coding consultant who works for Waldorf and Associates and is primarily responsible for coding the accounts from Walnut Grove Hospital. She has her own business associate agreement with Waldorf and Associates. Eloise's consulting business grew faster than she expected, so she subcontracted the work from Waldorf and Associates to Astor C. Elery but did not initiate a business associate agreement with her. Unfortunately, Astor was a victim of voice phishing (vishing) when, on April 2nd, she received what she thought was a legitimate call from the hospital's IT department wanting to verify her log-in credentials after a virus was detected. The caller, who presented himself as an IT representative, stated he needed the information in order to validate that the virus had not originated from her computer. Once the caller had Astor's access information, he was able to enter the hospital information system at will. He used it to locate the account of a prominent individual within the community, which included details about her recent venereal disease diagnosis. Two days after the vishing incident, the woman received a blackmail letter and immediately reported it to the police. They began an investigation to determine who the blackmailer was and from where the information had been obtained. That led them to the hospital and her primary care physician. After the hospital's IT department performed analysis of their system, it was clear the information had come from them, and specifically under the log-in of Astor.

1. From the evidence above, did a breach truly occur? Support your position.

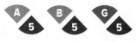

2. Consider the elements involved in this scenario and surmise which party is responsible for any notifications that must be made and support your position.

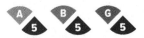

3. Based on the above information, will any notifications be necessary? Why or why not?

4. Present considerations for the hospitals IT system in the wake of this event. What types of system failures did this highlight in the hospital IT system?

References

AHIMA 2007 Privacy and Security Practice Council. 2008. How to React to a Security Incident. *Journal of AHIMA* 79(1): 66–70.

Brinda, D. and A. Watters. 2020. Data Privacy, Confidentiality, and Security. Chapter 11 in *Health Information Management: Concepts, Principles, and Practice*, 6th ed. P. Oachs and A. Watters, eds. Chicago: AHIMA.

Downing, K. 2014. Navigating a Compliant Breach Management Process. *Journal of AHIMA* 85(6): 56–58.

LeBlanc, M. 2020. Human Resources Management. Chapter 22 in *Health Information Management: Concepts, Principles, and Practice*, 6th ed. P. Oachs and A. Watters, eds. Chicago: AHIMA.

Reynolds, R. B. and M. S. Brodnik. 2017. The HIPAA Security Rule. Chapter 12 in *Fundamentals of Law for Health Informatics and Information Management*, 3rd ed. Chicago: AHIMA.

Rinehart-Thompson, L. A. 2017. HIPAA Privacy Rule: Part II. Chapter 11 in *Fundamentals of Law for Health Informatics and Information Management*, 3rd ed. M. S. Brodnik, L. A. Rinehart-Thompson, and R. B. Reynolds, eds. Chicago: AHIMA.

7.4 Merging and outsourcing transcription services

Competency VI.1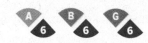

Competency VI.2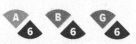

Maria is the new director of HIM at Beechwood City Hospital. This is her first director position. Upon her hire, she was directed to initiate a consolidation of transcription staff to include the radiology, pathology, and HIM transcriptionists. A consultant had determined that cross-training staff, implementing industry leading productivity standards for line count, and offering an incentive for achieving goals beyond the productivity standard would save the hospital over $150,000.00 per year.

Currently, each of the transcription groups, HIM, radiology, and pathology, have their own lead transcriptionist and different dictation system. Consolidating the services will result in just one lead position and create substantial savings. Additionally, the consultant found that based on the lines of dictation in all the departments and using the industry leading productivity standards, there were more transcriptionists than necessary in the organization. Merging the transcription services into one central service and increasing productivity would mean termination for a minimum of four full-time transcriptionists, again creating a cost savings. Finally, consolidating all transcription under one system will net an annual savings of $250,000 in software licenses, and maintenance.

Maria is reluctant to inform the transcription staff about the impending job losses for fear that many of the transcriptionists may be nervous enough to look for positions elsewhere leaving the hospital in a bind. She begins the process by informing all the transcriptionists of the merger and puts Gloria, her HIM lead transcriptionist, in charge of the combined team. Without sharing any of the rationale for her changes, Maria has the other two transcriptionists who were leads begin cross training of the staff to their specialties. She makes no change to their job status since they are performing the cross training, so no cost saving is realized. Gloria is put in charge of training radiologists and pathologists on the HIM dictation system.

Staff are slow to adapt to the differences in transcribing reports for radiology and pathology, so productivity decreases. Physicians are complaining about the lack of report availability in a timely manner. Meanwhile, the training of the radiologists and pathologists on the HIM system is also slow. Those physicians do not understand why there has to be a change and Gloria cannot answer their questions. Many of them continue to use the legacy system to dictate.

When Maria tries to implement the new productivity standards, the transcriptionists complain that the line count hasn't taken into consideration the hospital requirements that they must abide by. Work slows down even more.

At this point, backlog has grown and now Maria must outsource some of the transcription work. She finds a vendor who promises great turnaround time, excellent quality, and competitive pricing. After engaging with the vendor, it is clear that the vendor is able to handle this workload at a cost that is much lower than the in-house staff. Quality and turnaround time are being met as well. The chief financial officer (CFO) met with Maria and indicated that a decision had been made to outsource all transcription services beginning in one month.

1. Propose a better way that the initial transcription merger could have been handled by Maria by incorporating the change management process steps.

2. Present one factor that was a key element in the failure of the transcription merger and support your opinion.

3. Predict how this change process may have evolved differently if Maria had previous experience as a director.

4. Theorize how Maria could have used Gloria and the other lead transcriptionists to achieve the desired results in a more advantageous manner.

Reference

Shaw P. L. and D. Carter. 2019. *Quality and Performance Improvement in Healthcare: A Tool for Programmed Learning*, 7th ed. Chicago: AHIMA.

BUILDING A FUTURE CAREER?
YOU NEED THE RIGHT CREW!

You work hard to earn the skills and know-how you need for a job in health information management (HIM). Now lay a strong foundation with AHIMA membership at the affordable Student Member rate—of $49—almost 75% off active member dues!

AHIMA now bundles Student membership with a variety of textbooks and Virtual Lab. Ask your bookstore or professor and start saving!

JOIN NOW AND:

SUCCEED IN SCHOOL
- Merit Scholarships
- Digital *Journal of AHIMA*
- Body of Knowledge
- Engage Online Communities

PREPARE FOR A SUCCESSFUL CAREER
- Career Prep Webinars
- Salary Snapshot
- Mentor Match Program
- Career Prep Workbook
- *Career Minded* E-newsletter

GET A JOB
- Career Assist Job Bank
- AHIMA's Career Map
- Apprenticeship Program
- Virtual Career Fairs

CONNECT WITH OTHER HIM PROFESSIONALS
- Engage Online Communities
- Component State Association (CSA) Membership
- Student Academy at Convention
- Volunteer with AHIMA

SAVE MONEY ON
- Textbooks
- Certification Exams
- Meeting Registrations and More

Join today:

ahima.org/join

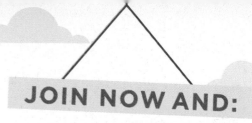

AHIMA
American Health Informati
Management Association